Blessed Hanna Chrzanowska, RN

A NURSE OF MERCY

GOSIA BRYKCZYŃSKA

Available from:
Marian Helpers Center
Stockbridge, MA 01263

Prayerline: 1-800-804-3823
Orderline: 1-800-462-7426

Websites: thedivinemercy.org
marian.org

Publication Date:
March 25, 2019
Solemnity of the Annunciation

Imprimi Potest:
Very Rev. Kazimierz Chwalek, MIC
Provincial Superior
The Blessed Virgin Mary, Mother of Mercy Province
March 25, 2019

Nihil Obstat:
Dr. Robert A. Stackpole, STD
Censor Deputatus

ISBN: 978-1-59614-501-6

Cover and page design: Curtis Bohner

All images from Catholic Association of Polish Nurses
and Midwives – Kraków Branch, unless otherwise noted.
Back cover photos by Marie Romagnano.

Printed in the United States of America

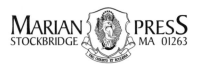

MARIAN PRESS
STOCKBRIDGE MA 01263

My work is not only my profession but also my vocation. A vocation which I have come to appreciate, as I fathom more deeply and internalise more particularly the words of Christ, I have come not to be served but to serve.

Hanna Chrzanowska

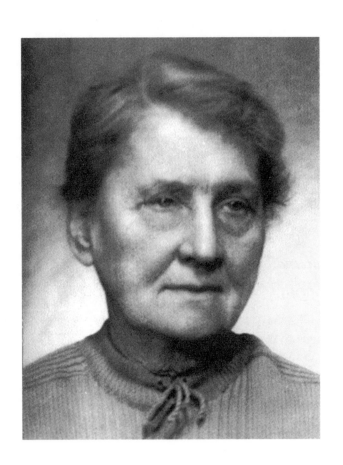

Acknowledgements

Many people have contributed to the writing of this book, and have helped me to improve the text. I would like especially to express my gratitude to Mme Helena Matoga, vice-postulator of the canonisation cause of Blessed Hanna Chrzanowska and members of the Kraków Branch of the *Catholic Nurses and Midwives Association*, without whose help and encouragement this extended biography of Hanna, the first such book to be written in English, would never have been produced.

It is difficult to write about the life of a woman whom you immensely admire but have never met personally; a woman who was, however, well known to my relatives, friends, colleagues and many acquaintances in Kraków and throughout Poland. I would therefore like to thank those many nurses and friends of Hanna, who have given me over many years, not only their permission to quote them and share their many reflections about Hanna, but who insisted that I should tell the world her wonderful story.

I would like to also thank many organizations and individuals for permission to use their photographs. *The Catholic Nurses and Midwives Association* in Kraków for materials and manuscripts from their archives, which are not available anywhere else and for their historical photographs, given to them by members of the Chrzanowski and Szlenkier families, with which to illustrate this biography. I would also like to especially thank Mr Stanislaw Szlenkier for his kind words of enthusiasm and encouragement. I wish to thank The Małopolska Regional Chamber of Nurses and Midwives for their continued help and support and for their historical photographs and the Polish Nursing Association (History of Nursing Section), especially Mme Krystyna Wolska-Lipiec, head of the Virtual Nursing Museum in Warsaw, for giving me access to their archives, photographs and those photographs bequeathed to them by alumni of the Warsaw School of Nursing. Likewise, I wish to thank the cloistered Dominican Nuns in

Kraków who graciously gave me several historical photos of the first school of nursing in Kraków, photos of Maria Epstein (Servant of God Sister Magdalena, OP) and to use photos from their own archives. I thank the Historical Museum of Kraków (Schindler's Factory), for photos of Kraków during the Second World War from their extensive and excellent collection. I would also like to thank the archivist at the Basilica of the Blessed Virgin Mary in Kraków, for permission to use the photo taken by Fr Gąsior, of the medieval crucifix carved by Wit Stworz. Many thanks to the Kraków University School of Nursing and The Parish of St Nicholas for having helped me in so many ways over the years.

The photos of activities relating to Parish nursing were taken by Sr Serafina Paluszek of the Sisters of St Felix, who was one of Hanna's earliest nursing co-workers in the Parish Nursing project. Photographs of Hanna Chrzanowska's funeral were by Mr Jerzy Rumun, and those of Hanna as a young girl and adolescent are all from family collections of the Chrzanowski and Szlenkier families now in the archives of the *Catholic Nurses and Midwives Association*, in Kraków. Finally I would like to thank the Benedictine community of Tyniec Abbey for photographs of Dom Piotr Rostworowski and Dom Placyd Galiński. I am also very grateful to the widow of Venerable Servant of God Jerzy Cisielski, Mme Danuta Cisielska, for permission to use a photograph of her husband.

I am also very grateful to Mr Russell McGuirk and Sr Elizabeth Rees for their editorial help in proof-reading, editing the text and suggestions for improvements. I wish to thank Marie Romagnano, RN, founder of Healthcare Professionals for Divine Mercy without whose enthusiasm and drive this manuscript would never have been published and for her photographs of the Beatification ceremony, shrine of Bl. Hanna in St Nicholas Church, Kraków and photos associated with the life of Bl Hanna. I also thank the Marian Fathers of the Immaculate Conception of the Blessed Virgin Mary in Stockbridge, MA who put so much trust in me and agreed to publish this book.

Finally, any responsibility for misrepresentation of facts or any mistakes that have crept into the book, in spite of all assistance and help, must lie solely with me.

Dr Gosia Brykczyńska, Pentecost 2018

CONTENTS

FOREWORD

It is an honour for me as President of the Comité International Catholique Infirmières et Assistants Médico-Sociales (CICIAMS) to write the foreword to this book of Hanna Chrzanowska's life and her road to sainthood. Hanna, a registered nurse, contributed to the formation of the Association of Catholic Union of Polish Nurses in 1937. She was a life-long member of the Kraków Branch of the Polish Association of Catholic Nurses which became affiliated with CICIAMS. It is indeed humbling to count Hanna, the first registered nurse to be beatified, as one of our own.

Hanna Chrzanowska's story is one that makes for compelling and inspiring reading and should be of interest to a wide variety of readers, particularly nurses, midwives and all involved in the health care and social professions and activities. It is a deeply spiritual, yet human, account of a professional, courageous and upright nurse, social activist, educator, manager, author, editor and legislator, who positively affected the lives of so many people often in the face of great opposition from civic authorities. It evokes many emotions such as awesome wonder, laughter, fear and inadequacy in the reader.

Hanna was a remarkable Polish citizen and patriot, a woman of many gifts and talents including a magnetism and spirituality that were wisely used. Her values were grounded in family roots of social consciousness, charitable works and philanthropic activities. Spanning the years 1902 to 1973, most of which were war-torn years in her country's history, she lived through the periods of occupation by Russians, followed by 20 years of independence, six years of horrors of the Second World War, and after that, it was back to occupation by Russian Socialist Communists, a period of Cold War and a time of suppression of Catholicism in all its forms. Born in Warsaw, the family moved to Kraków in 1912 where Hanna was to spend most of her life.

The author, Dr Gosia Brykczyńska, captures in a comprehensive way Hanna's life over the course of her 71 years. She maps out succinctly and clearly Hanna's journey including her personality, joys and sorrows from childhood through adolescence, general education and into adulthood. Considerable attention is given to her nurse education years, both basic and post-basic learning, in Poland, France, Belgium, and New York and her emerging and life-long interest in community and children's nursing, much of which is likely to resonate with the readers. Hanna's interactions with her family, friends, colleagues, clergy, local civic administrators, and national government are embraced and include examples of her pleasant countenance, wit, and joie de vivre. Her sufferings caused by the death of her father in a concentration camp, her brother and only sibling shot by the Russians, the death of a close friend, the death of an aunt, eviction of her mother and herself from their home during the Second World War make for poignant reading.

The account of Hanna's life includes detailed information regarding her professional work — nursing, teaching, managing, active membership in the Polish Professional Nursing Association, and her voluntary work with a wide variety of recipients such as the needy and poor, prisoners, refugees, displaced people, isolated, homeless, the disabled and other marginalised people; courageously, and often defiantly, undertaken during the times of German occupation, and later Communist rule. During the latter time, she was dismissed from her salaried position as a director of nursing as the result of her Catholic practices and moreover as the result of helping others to do likewise. Hanna was forced into premature retirement, after which she established Parish Nursing for people in their homes with the support of qualified nurses and volunteers from all walks of life. This ultimately successful project was aimed at meeting the nursing, social, and spiritual needs of individuals — irrespective of means and religious beliefs — not addressed by the then very limited government-controlled community nursing system. The establishment of such a system was not easy. Among those who enabled and encouraged Hanna in her dream in the early stages was the young Father Karl Wojtyla, later to become Pope Saint John Paul II.

There are also narratives of her spiritual life which became reflective and began to mature in her mid-30s and how, as it deepened, she integrated it in her daily life without ever being overtly religious. Her work, which she saw as a true vocation, mirrored the healing stories of the Gospels as evidenced by her interactions with the sick, housebound, and marginalised. She also brought spiritual solace to those requiring it through prayer, organising the celebration of Mass in their homes, and retreats under the auspices of such activities as holiday camps.

Dr Brykczyńska discusses Hanna's many interests. These included literature, theatre, music, and writing. Her writings were not only confined to numerous professional matters that included nursing legislation, community nursing, and training notes for volunteers. They also encompassed writing novels, some of which are semi-biographical, poetry, memoirs, newspaper articles, vignettes, and correspondences several of which are under the pseudonym of Agnieszka Osiecka.

Hanna's struggle with ill health throughout her whole life is outlined; including the diagnosis and treatment of gynaecological cancer in 1963 for which, when it returned in 1966, there was no further available treatment. Thereafter, she intensified her work, albeit from a less physical but more an administrative perspective, as she prepared herself for what she called 'the greatest adventure of all'.

There may be gaps in her story, especially those of a personal spiritual nature, as all Hanna's private papers and diaries were destroyed at her request upon her death. Suffice to say she responded to the nursing and social needs of her time with a spiritual fervour and work inextricably intertwined. Fortunately, there were records of some of her activities available from the Polish Association of Catholic Nurses and Midwives, her memoirs, semi-biographical novels, newspaper archives, and from those who knew her personally during her lifetime that enabled Dr Brykczyńska to relay this very credible account of Hanna's life. Of note are testimonies following the miraculous recovery of Hanna's friend and nurse, Zofia Szlendak-Cholewińska, from a non-medically treatable ruptured aneurysm of the brain. This miracle was attributed to Hanna's intercession and opened the way for her being declared Blessed by the Congregation of the Causes of Saints in the Vatican.

In conclusion, Dr Brykczyńska has managed very well to record the life of this remarkable nurse in a readable, honest, and engaging way by effectively weaving together differing aspects of Hanna's life to include her family, friends, nursing colleagues, volunteers, clergy, patients, the poor and needy, among others whose lives she touched, and indeed transformed in many cases. It should rank high in the recorded history of Hanna Chrzanowska's life.

Ora et Labora

Geraldine McSweeney
International President CICIAMS
Dublin
March 2018

A Note from the Sponsor: Healthcare Professionals for Divine Mercy

The moment I discovered that a lay registered nurse, Hanna Chrzanowska, was announced to be beatified, I wished to know everything about her. The more I read, the more I realized how faithfully she lived out her vocation to serve Christ by caring for the sick and the dying. She was an extraordinary nurse that performed her duties out of deep love for the sick. Relying on Christ, insurmountable difficulties — including lifelong illness — did not deter her from working tirelessly to overcome the desperate, neglected conditions of the sick in her community.

At her Beatification on April 28, 2018, I was privileged to carry one of the small lit oil lamps in procession. I was filled with joy that a lay nurse who embraced and encountered Christ in the sick as her vocation, and placed before all the faithful an outstanding example of Christian service was being raised to the honors of the altar. The Healthcare Professionals for Divine Mercy, an apostolate of the Marian Fathers of the Immaculate Conception, which I represent as its Founder and Director, is sponsoring this first Marian Press edition of *Blessed Hanna Chrzanowska: A Nurse of Mercy*. The National Shrine of The Divine Mercy in Stockbridge, Massachusetts, which already serves as the spiritual center of devotion to St. Faustina and Blessed Michael Sopocko in America will also include Blessed Hanna Chrzanowska as its newest witness to Divine and human mercy.

I wish to thank Gosia Brykczyńska, PhD, RN, OCV for writing this biography of Blessed Hanna and for allowing me to assist in this publication. I also wish to thank Very Rev. Kazimierz Chwalek, MIC for his dedication and support. I also thank M. Scott Nelson, RN, BSN who served as proofreader. As a publication director, I wish to thank the Congregation of Sisters of Our Lady of Mercy and Małgorzata Pabis for permission to use photos from the beatification of Blessed Hanna.

I ask Blessed Hanna to intercede for the Healthcare Professionals for Divine Mercy and especially for Nurses for Divine Mercy and become the special patron for the members of these groups. It is my hope that that each nurse and healthcare professional will take to heart this extraordinary woman's life as a nurse and learn that holiness is an achievable reality when keeping one's eyes on Christ.

Marie F. Romagnano, RN, BSN, CRC, CCM
Founder, Healthcare Professionals for Divine Mercy

A NURSE OF MERCY

INTRODUCTION

There are many wonderful holy women, and some of them, in answering the call to follow Christ, manage to do amazing things. Their heroic Christian lives witness to the power and glory of the risen Lord, spreading love and joy whenever and wherever their story is retold. This is the story about one such woman, who went about her ordinary professional tasks as a registered community nurse-teacher in a most extraordinary, Christ-centred way.

The story I present to the reader is about a pioneering Polish nurse, Hanna Chrzanowska (1902–1973) who, as a lay Catholic woman, worked for most of her professional life as a qualified instructor in the field of community nursing. She established and coordinated Parish Nursing in Communist Poland during the darkest days of the Cold War; and it is for this work that she is especially remembered, by the grateful people of Kraków.

She was also a great Polish patriot, and during the Second World War her tireless work with refugees, on behalf of Cardinal Sapieha's Benevolence Committee, significantly contributed to the avoidance of mass homelessness, hunger, and outright starvation in the overcrowded city. She was a talented, highly intelligent and gracious woman, full of zest for life, and with a legendary sense of humour. There is no doubt that she had been endowed with many personal gifts, talents, and social advantages, but she also managed to give back to society, the nursing world, and her faith community far more than she ever received.

To support her innovative nursing spirituality, she became a Benedictine oblate of Tyniec Abbey. Becoming a Benedictine oblate helped to raise Hanna's already deep sense of the Divine and not insignificant involvement in Catholic activism, to a whole new level of spiritual engagement. Hanna was already a devout practising Catholic who saw herself as being 'single for the Lord'; the oblature commitment encouraged and sustained her unequivocal following of Christ, which she did with a gospel-based zeal and single-mindedness, as is required of a serious disciple of St Benedict.

Hanna's life superbly illustrated the Benedictine motto *Ora et Labora – Work and Pray*. She worked hard and conscientiously and prayed fervently and meaningfully and was known to play and relax with great abandon, appreciating all that life had to offer. She lived almost half of her life in times of war and economic hardship and during the harsh Communist era which followed. Her nursing spirituality reflects these stark realities. Hers was no sugar-coated devotional approach to religion, but a firmly feet-on-the ground joyful acquiescence to the will and love of God. While she had no great mystical moments, or at least none that we know of, her life was clearly marked out with the obvious interventions and supportive love of Christ. She was also surrounded and supported, in a most extraordinary and visible way, by a veritable community and communion of saints. She did not become who she was destined to be, with the help of Divine Grace, in isolation.

Some of the saints who surrounded Hanna have now been formally recognised as such by the church, including Pope St John Paul II; and her three friends whose canonisation causes have been opened: Maria Epstein (Sister Maria Magdalena, OP), Janina Woynarowska, a nurse, and the Warsaw-based social worker Teresa Strzembosz, as well as the engineer Jerzy Ciesielski, now declared 'Venerable', who worked as a volunteer with students in Hanna's community project. All these people have already been recognised by the Church as having lived exemplary Christian lives and worthy to be considered for sainthood. But there were also many unsung, quiet, and invisible saints who worked alongside Hanna, often for years, and who make up a far longer list. People such as Hanna's close friend and co-worker Maria Starowiejska, and her nursing colleague Aleksandra Dąmbska, or Hanna's assistant in the Parish nursing project and fellow Benedictine oblate, Alina Rumun. All these "saints" supported and helped Hanna to become the holy woman she really was, through their tangible and intangible assistance — professionally and also through friendship — including prayer, example, and a similar dedication to committed Christian service.

Sadly, there is still a conviction, among many Catholics, that to be considered a real, that is, an efficacious Saint, you need to have been dead for least a couple of hundred years. This curious time-related distancing of oneself from the life of a saint may be reduced however, if during the saint's lifetime they were known to be a mystic, with accompanying levitations, bi-locations and/or visions and miracle-performing gifts, or if they were simply considered to be larger than life — like Mother Teresa of Calcutta. Otherwise, a passage of several centuries is considered a good measure of saintly maturity. This hagiographic truism is borne out by the continuing and endearing cults of St Anthony of Padua, or St Rita, or St Francis of Assisi, to name but a few. In more recent times the great miracle-performing Capuchin friar St Padre Pio or the humble Polish sister St Faustyna, engage many millions of Catholics in devotional activities. Saints whose lives did not manifest extraordinary supernatural gifts, who during their life on earth worked as mere professionals or farmers, or factory workers or even ran homeless shelters and soup kitchens as did Dorothy Day, just don't come close to that level of universal recognition of sanctity.

For most people, the notion that the doctor in the local hospital, the butcher down the road, or the newly-arrived young priest in the parish could be a saint — is unthinkable, almost sacrilegious. Somehow, anyone we could possibly know, can never, by definition, be holy enough to be considered a potential saint. We put saints on a pedestal which is so high that no-one can even see the top of the plinth. It is therefore not at all clear who can actually stand upon the sainthood plinth and who we would even want to place there. And yet, ordinary physicians have been declared saints, as have butchers, bakers, and bridge-builders. Heaven, we are told by the Church, even contains a goodly number of young seminarians and newly ordained priests, who were often martyrs, but not always. In fact, heaven is full of people just like us — butchers, bakers and candlestick makers, and even nurses. Yet it comes as a surprise, when we read the life of a person who lived 'in our times', and who it is suggested, lived a life worthy of being considered a model of Christian virtue, i.e., of being a saint. And yet we are all encouraged, in fact commanded, to become saints — to live as saints. It is also a strange truth, that many so-called

great saints were not necessarily perceived as such during their lifetime, or at least not by everyone, such as the young Carmelite, St
Thérèse of Lisieux.

It is not my intention to expand here on the doctrine of the
communion of saints or to comment on the regulations and guidelines
governing the elevation of souls to the ranks of sainthood — but I
think that it is worth reflecting on some of these issues, in the context
of getting to know the life and works of Hanna Chrzanowska. We
know that in the past few decades, starting with the pontificate of
Pope St John Paul II, the veils of secrecy and bureaucracy have been
gradually stripped away from the Roman offices of The Congregation for the Causes of Saints, making it much easier now to navigate
officialdom. We also know that far more good Christians have been
beatified and canonised in this last half-century, than ever before. Just
a year ago in July 2017, Pope Francis reaffirmed this, decreeing in his
Moto Proprio *Maiorem Hac Dilectionem* that to give up your life for
another, as an act of charity, as might be the case in rescuing someone
from danger or to save their life, can be considered a sufficient reason,
among the obvious requirements for evidence of piety, to open a cause
for canonisation (in Latin – *oblatio vitae*). This could well become the
case with the Polish Ulma family, who harboured Jews during the Second World War and were all killed as a consequence of this, by Nazi
soldiers in 1944.

That Hanna is considered an exemplary pioneer of nursing in
Poland, is an undeniable fact. She was one of the first young women in
Poland to attend a nursing school and become a registered nurse, and
her extremely active professional life is the subject of very many articles and chapters in books on the history of nursing in Poland and in
Central Europe. Even if she were never proclaimed a saint, she would
still be considered a remarkable woman who did much to promote her
chosen profession and to alleviate suffering among her patients. In
fact, her colleagues, friends, and patients saw more in her than just the
reflection of a good, competent, even an extraordinary nurse. But just
what did they see in her and how did they assess Hanna's life, in order
to reach the conclusion that she was not only a founding member of
the nursing profession in Poland, but more to the point that she was a
special soul, a Christian example for all, a saint?

When recounting the life of a saint it is always good to remember to ground their activities and apostolate in the context of their times. I have consciously tried to achieve this while writing this biography, and I have deliberately kept both the names of people and places intact and in full as explicitly as possible, with dates where appropriate, in order to facilitate further research and investigation into Hanna's times and activities by those English language readers who may not have easy access to Polish archival material, or even possess a full knowledge of recent central European history. As we know, people become saints by living to the full and engaging with others, not by just passively existing here on earth. They live at a particular time and in a particular place, fulfilling their duties and commitments to the best of their abilities, for the love of God and in accordance with His will. They are people belonging to their specific historical period and country; they are not some timeless phantoms floating around an indeterminate universe. They live their Christ-centred lives as well as they can, and they do this never forgetting who they really are, where they are going to, and who awaits them at the end of the day.

One of the biggest problems I have encountered, when promoting Hanna's beatification, has been the difficulty of demonstrating to well-intentioned doubters that simply being a good and conscientious nurse can indeed become a pathway to heaven, and that fulfilling the role of a nurse — for the love of Christ — can enable the healthcare worker to become a saint, that is, a person fit for heaven. Nursing for the committed Christian, (like any other job, in fact), must become an activity fit and appropriate for a saint. Otherwise something is out of sync. At times we may have to adapt our work to sanctify it — but all human work, whether in shops, in offices, in hospitals, or railway stations, can, should, and in fact must enable us to become saints. That, and a healthy dose of humour.

Hanna's most profound spiritual moments were as intimate and private as was the rest of her personal life. Few were privileged to know or were privy to her innermost thoughts, or were able to look into the depth of her spirituality, but all could experience the fruits of her living, vibrant faith and prayer-filled life. There was a clarity of Christ-focused intention about her nursing, which was present for all to appreciate. In spite of the fact that all her personal papers were burnt immediately after her death, following Hanna's explicit request, enough material has fortunately survived, because it was already in the public domain, for us to gain at least a small glimpse of her beautiful Benedictine nursing spirituality. Hanna quietly and discreetly lived out the evangelical call to ease suffering and pain, and to recognise Christ in the stranger; and she did this all the while working as a community nursing instructor and later as co-ordinator of parish nurses in the most difficult circumstances.

The opening of Hanna's cause for canonisation in 1995 was requested of Cardinal Franciszek Macharski by none other than her own nursing colleagues and students: apparently a first for the Vatican records. The canonisation process itself proceeded extremely quickly, bearing in mind that Hanna was a lay person who was neither a martyr nor a religious or even a member of an established Church movement. The Catholic nurses of Kraków took over the care of the case. Even the Vice-postulator for the cause, Mme. Helena Matoga, had been one of Hanna's nursing students. Soon, almost forty-five years to the day from the date of her death, Hanna will be formally counted by the Church among the many holy women in heaven known for their works of mercy and for their care of the sick and abandoned.

It is to be hoped that Blessed Hanna will become a patron saint and model for today's generation of Benedictine oblates, nurses, social workers and for all those who work professionally as volunteers with and for the sick, the elderly and the chronically ill: those people who are still marginalised by our society today and who are still forgotten and abandoned. As Christ said, 'the poor you will always have among you' (Mt.26.11), so there will always be room for love and mercy to triumph as it did when Hanna was alive and she visited the homes of her patients in Kraków.

CHAPTER 1

Uncovering the Past:
Family Roots and Historical Background

'All things must come to the soul from its roots,
from where it is planted.'

— St Teresa of Avila

It was late afternoon, but the small chapel of the Discalced Carmelite nuns on Łobzowska Street in Kraków was full to overflowing. Chairs had been put out on the pavement in front of the chapel to accommodate the large crowds of elderly people who had gathered outside. Passers-by on their way home from work were surprised to see so many elderly wheelchair-bound mourners, attended by young student nurses, and the sheer variety and number of religious sisters and brothers all in their different habits, not to mention the significant presence of university students and professors. It appeared that people from all over Kraków, indeed from everywhere in Poland, had come to attend a funeral Mass. Crowds like this were most unusual in those hard Communist times; obviously this was no ordinary funeral Mass.

Not only was the local parish priest present but also many other priests from the city of Kraków, with a few *Monsignori* from the Bishop's palace, together with Bishop Franciszek Macharski, representing the diocese. Most amazing of all, Cardinal Karol Wojtyła (now Pope St John II) was presiding over the solemn liturgy. Curious passers-by asked which of the Carmelite nuns had recently died, only to be told that this was a funeral Mass not for one of the nuns but for a nurse, named Hanna Chrzanowska.

Such were the recollections of Maria Dawidowska-Strzembosz, a friend and colleague of Hanna, (also sister-in-law of Hanna's close friend and collaborator Teresa Strzembosz – but more about them later), who attended that funeral in Kraków in the spring of 1973. What Maria remembered most was the enormous crowd of handicapped, frail and elderly mourners. At a time when the old and infirm, the wheelchair-bound and disabled were kept at home behind closed doors, this was an extraordinary show of social and moral defiance. But all these otherwise housebound individuals had once been Hanna's patients, and they were present in the monastery chapel that spring day to say goodbye and thank you, one last time, for all she had done for them.

Such a palpable and moving demonstration of affection and respect is rare and requires some explanation, for Hanna Chrzanowska was indeed no ordinary woman, no ordinary nurse. In the historic Rakowicki cemetery of Kraków, engraved on her original tombstone was the simplest of inscriptions: *Hanna Chrzanowska – daughter of Ignacy and Wanda Chrzanowska*. Today her body lies in an alabaster sarcophagus in the church of St Nicholas, in the hospital district of Kraków, and added to her name is the word 'Pielęgniarka' — nurse. That short word encapsulates the whole of Hanna Chrzanowska's life, work and personality. In order, therefore, to relate the narrative of her life and describe the nature of her extraordinary pastoral work, and in so doing to illustrate her caring and saintly wisdom, it is necessary first to place her in an historical context.

By any standards Hanna was an exceptional woman, but one who nonetheless was a fairly typical product of her socio-economic background and times. The Chrzanowski family came from the Podlasie region of eastern Poland, and Hanna's father, Ignacy Chrzanowski, came from an impoverished but highly patriotic family of landed gentry. In keeping with many similar families in the then Russian-occupied part of Poland, they were severely restricted in their social and cultural activities by successive edicts of Tsars, following a series of abortive uprisings and revolts, in particular the doomed patriotic uprising of 1863. This uprising resulted in huge social upheavals among the landed gentry, many of whom found their lands confiscated and their traditional means of livelihood severely curtailed. As a result, many young men and women from this hitherto privileged social class turned in even greater numbers than before to various professions and to business ventures as a source of alternative income. In the partitioned Poland of the final years of the nineteenth century, these new professionals, joining the ranks of the already well-established middle-class *intelligentsia*, represented a powerful, highly influential, and patriotic new elite.

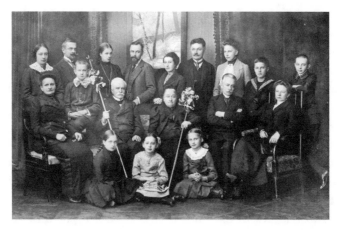

The Chrzanowski family attending the wedding anniversary of Hanna's grandparents. Hanna is sitting on the ground first from the right.

Hanna's father was related on his mother's side to the famous Polish writer Henryk Sienkiewicz, who in 1905 received the Nobel Prize in Literature for his fictional portrayal of the lives of early Christians in his acclaimed novel *Quo Vadis*. In her memoirs, Hanna recalls visits to the house of this notable and much-loved relative. Hanna's paternal grandparents belonged to the landed gentry and were known for their patriotism, deep religious convictions and genuine admiration of scholarship. Her father was sent to the best schools in Warsaw, Breslau (today Wrocław in Western Poland) and Berlin. In 1895 having finished his university courses, he settled in Warsaw, where he taught Polish language and literature and conducted covert seminars which were quickly made illegal by the Tsar. He also helped to set up Literacy Schools for poor children. He was a democrat with liberal inclinations.

Although Ignacy Chrzanowski was not a practising Catholic as a young adult, this attitude changed somewhat as he became older, for his graduate students in Kraków remember seeing him on more than one occasion praying in the town's medieval basilica; and his wife,

Wanda Szlenkier commented in her journal that as a mature man he was a person for whom God and concerns of the faith mattered a lot. But he was not a rigorously practising Catholic. He was an admirer of Rudolf Steiner. He did not suffer fools gladly, but he was prepared to champion many difficult causes, which got him into trouble with the authorities on more than one occasion. Above all, he was passionate about the arts and music, and especially Polish literature. To this day he is fondly remembered for his seminal textbook on Polish literature, which was published in 1908; a textbook that has since become a much loved classic, having gone through countless editions and revisions, and which is still in print.

Many spoke of him as a man of truth, enormous energy, and great goodness. Hanna noted in her memoirs that the goodness of her father was almost a miraculous goodness "... and was the natural continuation of the great goodness to be found in the home of my paternal grandparents. This goodness shone in its own particular way, with a sparkle lavishly thrown at it by God, with a generosity known only to God. It was a goodness expressed specifically towards the next person, concretely, one's neighbour...." In the lifestyle, preferences, and choices that Hanna made as a mature woman, one can see the reflection of her father, a person who profoundly inspired and shaped her personality.

At the turn of the nineteenth century and for much of the duration of the Second Polish Republic, over a third of the inhabitants of Poland belonged to various ethnic minority groups and professed a variety of religious allegiances. This rich heterogeneous cultural and religious legacy has been almost entirely lost in modern Poland after the horrors and ethnic cleansing of the Second World War and following the 1946 Potsdam Agreement which radically re-drew the boundaries of post-war Poland. But for Poles in the 1900s, interfaith marriages would have been fairly common. On the 4 November 1899, in a highly publicised social wedding in Warsaw, Dr Ignacy Chrzanowski married Wanda Szlenkier, the daughter of Lutheran entrepreneurs and philanthropists.

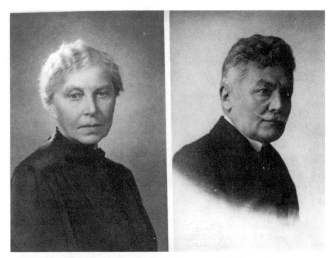

Wanda Szlenkier and Ignacy Chrzanowski, Hanna's parents.

Wanda Szlenkier was the daughter of Maria and Karol Szlen-kier, both rich citizens of Warsaw. Their palatial home in Warsaw is today the official residence of the Italian Embassy. Hanna wrote in her memoirs that her maternal grandfather made his fortune through his own hard work, cautiously adding that her grandfather's employ-ees probably had a better life than many self-employed businessmen. Notwithstanding the fact that this comment was written by Hanna at the height of the Communist repression, it gives an interesting insight into Hanna's opinion of her grandfather's relations with his employees. Hanna's maternal grandfather, apart from providing employment for many individuals, also established and maintained a Technical School for young artisans; and Maria Szlenkier, her maternal grandmother, helped set up a health centre for poor children in Warsaw. Hanna commented about her maternal grandparents that they were 'the most authentic of philanthropists. I grew up in an atmosphere of service to one's neighbour and so-called 'charity-work' — as if this were the most natural (and normal) of attitude.'

Hanna's mother, like her father, was a powerful and influential figure in the development of Hanna's personality. While enjoying her status in the community, Wanda never forgot those less fortunate than herself. She had a quick and perceptive mind which saw and registered much and was capable of analysing situations methodically.

She was a supportive mother to Hanna but never overly protective —
an attitude which would only have smothered Hanna's lively and free
spirit. Her example of magnanimity and largesse was mirrored in the
exuberant graciousness and generosity displayed by Hanna. Hanna
was very much, therefore, the child of her parents, and she was often
heard to comment that she felt proud and indeed privileged to be
their daughter.

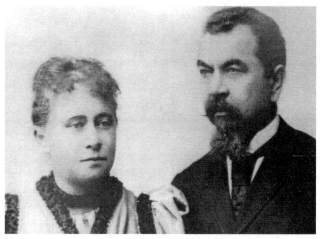

Hanna's maternal grandparents – Maria and Karol Szlenkier

Hanna's maternal aunt, Zofia Szlenkier, was also a well-known
Polish philanthropist, who in 1913 founded and endowed a paedi-
atric hospital in Warsaw, the Mary and Charles Hospital (*Szpital
Imienia Marii i Karola*), named after Hanna's maternal grandparents.
Aunt Zofia was an immensely significant person in the life of young
Hanna, for it was she who was instrumental in establishing the first
professional school of nursing in Poland, in 1924. However, before
her involvement with that school in Warsaw, she first went abroad to
Geneva to train as a physician, but sadly she was unable to complete
her studies, as she had to return to Poland due to family commitments. Later, as a still relatively young woman of twenty-five, she was
accepted to train as a nurse at St Thomas' Hospital School of Nursing
in London, where she had the good fortune to meet the aged, and
by then somewhat frail, Florence Nightingale. But she was unable to

complete this training either — although at least she now had some idea of what was expected of a trained nurse.

Hanna recalled that for her Aunt Zofia, to take on the role of a nursing probationer in London as a mature, independent woman, financially secure, and having already endowed a major paediatric hospital, must have demanded self-denial and dogged determination. But Zofia Szlenkier wanted to be a *real nurse*, that is, a trained and qualified nurse (after the English fashion), and therefore she was prepared to work hard to achieve that goal. She did not want to be a Director of Nurses, responsible for running an exemplary paediatric hospital, without being a qualified nurse herself. Eventually in 1929, she was to become the Nursing Director of the newly founded Warsaw School of Nursing. Hanna's personality and motivations in life owed much to the forward-thinking and enlightened vision of this energetic, charismatic, and favourite aunt.

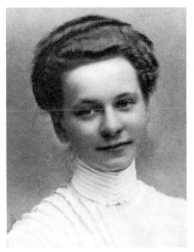

Zofia Szlenkier, Hanna's maternal aunt

Meanwhile, Hanna's mother abandoned the idea of building as she put it 'her own orphanage'— a dream which she had cherished for some time — and decided to put her not insignificant resources and efforts into supporting the existing paediatric hospital founded by her younger sister. This joint effort at thoughtful philanthropy was to be a notable characteristic of the Szlenkier family.

Chapter 2

The Land of Childhood: Early Years in Warsaw

'That great Cathedral space which was childhood.'
— Virginia Woolf

Wanda and Ignacy Chrzanowski had two children, a son Bohdan, born in 1900, and Hanna, born on 7 October 1902, and baptised on 23 July 1903 in the parish church of St Wojciech (Adalbert) in Wiązownia, near Warsaw, where the Szlenkiers had their impressive summer manor house. In keeping with all birth and christening certificates from that part of partitioned Poland, Hanna's official documents were written in Russian, which was to cause problems for her later, during the 1939-45 war, when she needed to prove to the occupying Soviet army her *Polish* nationality.

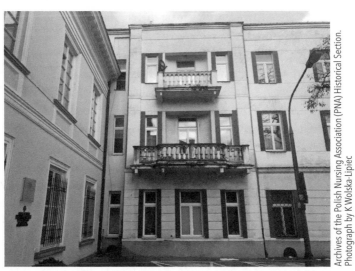

Archives of the Polish Nursing Association (PNA) Historical Section.
Photograph by K Wolska-Lipiec

Apartment in Warsaw on Senatorska Street where Hanna was born.

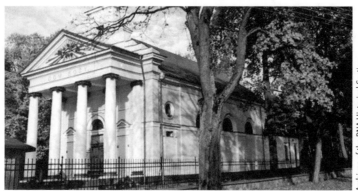

Archives of the PNA Historical Section.
Photograph by R. Szczęsny.

Church of St Wojciech (Adalbert) in Wązownia outside Warsaw
where Hanna was baptised.

Hanna's early childhood was spent mostly in Warsaw with her maternal grandparents. During longer holidays she also visited her paternal grandparents on their estate in Podlasie, in eastern Poland, an experience which left her with many happy memories. Years later, Hanna was to remember those carefree, sun-filled summers in Podlasie, nostalgically recalling '...Podlasie, with its meadows, birch groves and thickets of alder... [But] I will not delve into the black mesh of alder thicket through the rosy eyelets of which can be seen the setting sun. I will not pause to rest by the gardener's shed, or even by the avenue of linden-trees, or linger by the charming little manor house with its tiled stove in the salon....'

Hanna's childhood was undoubtedly privileged, sheltered and idyllic, with many delightful and fun-filled episodes; and it is to Hanna's credit that she did not waste those happy opportunities which life presented to her. In her memoirs she recalls an episode with a naughty but favourite dachshund belonging to her maternal grandmother, a dog called *Dar* (which means "gift" in Polish). The little dog realised that the softest and most comfortable place in the entire house in which to curl up and sleep undisturbed was on his mistress's *priedieu*, much to the annoyance and horror of the elderly lady. In recounting this story and many others like it, Hanna demonstrates a lively sense of humour and ever-present sense of joy — a sense of fun at the silly and often idiotic things that life throws our way. She could see the funny side of life and would laugh heartily at amusing idiosyncrasies.

Even more importantly, in her childhood and adult life she was always capable of enjoying her own foibles and peculiarities. All her life she was known to be an essentially joyful person, capable of infectious laughter and quick wit.

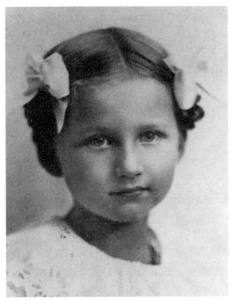

Young Hanna

Although she experienced a model childhood, she was aware from an early age that idyllic conditions such as hers were not shared by many of her young contemporaries. She recalls in her memoirs a particular instance from her childhood. While hospitalised with German measles in her Aunt Zofia's Children's Hospital in Warsaw, she noticed a poor boy who had no clothes in which to go home. Presumably, the "rags" in which he had been admitted to the hospital had been disposed of. Hanna was allowed to arrange for a new set of clothes for the boy and was told that she could be present when he was discharged home in the clothes that she had helped to organise for him. Hanna notes that this was an excellent pedagogical approach on the part of her aunt for teaching young Hanna about charity and relief-work since, as she observed, she was involved in the entire process from beginning to end.

This was not a form of depersonalised almsgiving from a safe distance, but direct help to a very real person who was in need. The young Hanna could immediately see the benefit (and effects) of her intervention. According to Hanna, in order to be authentic, true help for a specific person ought *not* to be anonymous. There is a place for anonymous giving (usually money) to good works and projects, but there is also the human need for genuine dialogue between the helper and the person in need of help. It is not too difficult to see in this childhood experience the lasting effects on Hanna's activities as an adult.

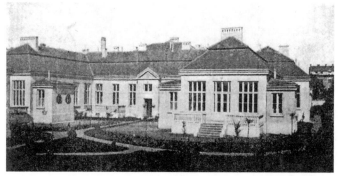

Hospital founded by Zofia Szlenkier – *Karol and Maria* –
where Hanna was a patient as a young girl.

As a child Hanna studied privately at home, often having to interrupt her schooling to take extended health-breaks — usually in the Tatra Mountains. She did not have robust health. While never considering herself an invalid, and able to maintain a prodigious professional output, she did experience lifelong health problems, most notably those associated with respiratory and immunological deficiencies. In time, going up to the mountains would become not only a health measure but also a chosen passion and a deliberate act of quiet, prayerful retreat.

As a young woman, and up to the time of her death, she found relaxation and joy through walking along mountain trails, and she did this regularly throughout the year, not only in the summer months. She delighted in the scenery and the natural world, especially in the variety of plants and small animals, learning their names and habits. She also greatly enjoyed sharing this knowledge with others. Her close friends recall the seriousness with which she approached the identification of plants and the pocket-sized nature book which she took with her wherever she went, so that she and others could identify plants. This deep appreciation of the physical world and amazement at the intricacies of creation and her wonder, therefore, at the indescribable magnificence of its creator, was all a form of prayer for Hanna; something which she pointed out to her friends and acquaintances, at every opportunity.

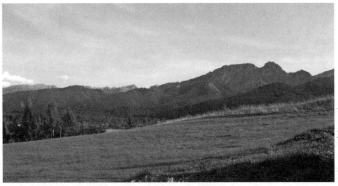

The Polish Tatra Mountains

Once, while accompanying a handicapped adolescent on a long train journey from Kraków to Laski, a retreat centre outside Warsaw, Hanna sat quietly observing the young woman reading her prayers from a book, head lowered over the pages of small print. She watched for a while and then decided to intervene, saying quite firmly, 'Close the prayer-book and start looking out of the window — there is the source of your real prayer of thanksgiving….' It should be added that the young woman had only shortly before that train trip left her flat for the first time, after many years of being unable to leave it. Due to the interventions of Hanna's Parish nurses, she was now being introduced to a new world outside the walls of her apartment, and therefore looking at and admiring nature from a train window would have been something completely novel for her.

Meanwhile, Hanna's recurrent bad health meant that she not only spent time recuperating in the Polish mountains, but that she was also sent abroad to sanatoria in Germany, Switzerland and southern France. This early exposure to foreign cultures and languages partly explains her excellent linguistic abilities, which were to become so useful in later life. Subsequently she would use her experiences in the sanatoria as a basis for the semi-autobiographical novels which she wrote and published in the 1930s, especially her last one, Blazing Snow (*Płonący Śnieg*), which is based on a sanatorium in Davos, Switzerland.

In 1910, Hanna's father was appointed professor of Polish language and literature at the Jagiellonian University in Kraków. This was a great honour for the young academic and the whole family moved to Kraków, a place where, with a few breaks, Hanna was to spend the rest of her life. The significance of Kraków to patriotic Poles at that time cannot be overestimated. Kraków had been the medieval capital of Poland. To this day, it is full of wonderful Romanesque and Gothic buildings and is dominated by an ancient fortified castle and cathedral, known as *The Wawel*, where many Polish kings and notables are buried.

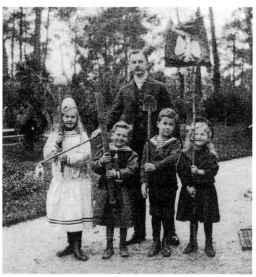

Young patriot Hanna holding a banner with the Polish emblem of a white eagle (first on the right) next to her is her brother Bohdan and their cousins. Standing behind them is Hanna's uncle.

For Hanna's family, the move to Kraków was also highly significant as the University — known as the Jagiellonian University after its early benefactors, Prince Władysław Jagiełło of Lithuania and his wife, Królowa Jadwiga (Queen Hedwige) — was the second oldest in central Europe; it represented learning and tradition. It was founded in 1364 and over the following centuries developed a well-deserved reputation as a centre of academic excellence and scholarship.

For young patriotic Poles prior to the outbreak of World War I, Kraków was an attractive town in which to live. The Austro-Hungarian authorities, who were governors of that section of partitioned Poland known as Galicia, allowed the Poles much self-governance, the use of the Polish language in schools and public places, and most importantly, allowed Polish to be the official language of the university. This meant that the Jagiellonian University was the *only* university in partitioned Poland where Polish was the accepted official language for academic studies.

At the beginning of the twentieth century, Kraków was also a haven for elderly, exiled partisans and insurrectionists who had been barred from returning to Russian-occupied Poland, having served their prison sentence in exile in Siberia for participating in the January 1863 insurrection. It was also the place of choice for Poles fleeing from political and economic hardship in Prussian-occupied western Poland. Kraków, therefore, was not only a centre of learning, but also a focus for patriotic fervour, a place with an atmosphere conducive to artistic endeavour and, last but not least, a place of relative religious tolerance and freedom.

The Imperial Austrian Governorship of Galicia exercised religious tolerance and allowed the expression of local Catholic and Jewish piety. Up to the Second World War, Kraków had a large, vibrant Jewish population, living mainly in a section of the town called Kazimierz, after King Kazimierz the Great who allowed Jews in 1335, who had been expelled from other parts of Europe or who were already living around Kraków, to legally settle across the river from the Royal castle, and to live and work in this royal city. But today there are only a few synagogues left and almost no resident Jews, as the majority of the pre-war population did not survive the horrors of the Holocaust. But in 1910 Kraków, the provincial capital of western Galicia, boasted many beautiful synagogues and of course churches (including Protestant chapels), and a proliferation of newly established religious congregations and orders — since only in Galicia were such faith-related activities allowed to flourish and to expand legitimately. Not surprisingly,

Kraków was referred to by some observers as the Rome of Central Europe. The combined effect of such cultural and religious freedom on Galicia as a whole, and in particular on the city of Kraków, was that more than anywhere else in partitioned Poland, the inhabitants felt free to be Poles, albeit lacking full political sovereignty. The eight-year-old Hanna arrived here at the beginning of the school year.

Initially Hanna continued her private lessons at home, but in 1912 she was enrolled in a private, co-educational, non-denominational, experimental school run by Miss Stanisława Okołowicz.

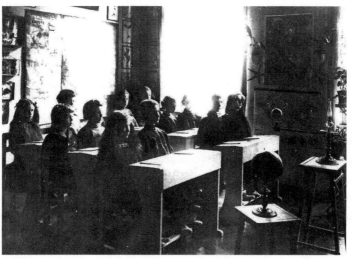

Hanna sitting at her desk by the window in Miss Okołowicz's school.

This school was highly unusual for those times, and its choice for Hanna reflected her parents' liberal educational attitudes in general and the teaching methods preferred by her father. The staff at the school consisted of some of the greatest names in Polish education and pedagogy, all great linguists and great patriots. In 1913 however, Hanna's formal education was to be disrupted yet again by her need to convalesce in Zakopane, a resort in the Tatra Mountains, with a teacher to accompany her.

The outbreak of the Great War in 1914 found Hanna staying with her maternal grandparents outside Warsaw. Unable to return to Kraków because the Front Line separated her from the rest of the family, she spent the intervening year being schooled privately in Warsaw. During this enforced stay in Warsaw she fell ill with German measles, requiring a stay in her Aunt Zofia's paediatric hospital. These early, positive, experiences of hospital care profoundly affected her opinion about nursing and healthcare work as an adult. Years later she observed that the experience only intensified her resolve to work in a hospital as a nurse. Hanna considered this experience of staying in hospital to be a pivotal moment in her social and moral development. She made the interesting comment in her memoirs that, had she been writing fiction and not an account of her life, she would have based the central character of her novel on the real-life nurse who looked after her in hospital. But Hanna was not so taken in by the starched uniforms and the hallowed aura of the institution that she could not detect flaws in the system. She clearly saw the difference between the care given by kind and efficient nurses and physicians, and that given by individuals who lacked warmth and consideration. Indeed, she says in her autobiography that she resolved then and there never to follow the example of a particularly uncaring physician.

Every minute of the hospital stay seems to have been encoded in her memory, and she apparently forgot no detail of the episode, from the various people who looked after her, right down to the design on the patterned wall-paper frieze in the hospital room where she was staying, and her sheer delight at seeing colourful children's characters from fairy tales painted on the tiles along the corridors. Years later Hanna recalled that the tiles in the Warsaw hospital were modeled on those in the children's ward at St Thomas' Hospital in London. When Hanna's Aunt Zofia was studying nursing in London at that English hospital, she was so captivated by these colourful tiles that she brought examples of them back with her to Poland and had similar ones mounted in the children's hospital which she had endowed. Moreover, the original English tiles which Hanna's aunt had seen at St Thomas' Hospital, can still be admired by visitors today.

CHAPTER 3

A Richness of Memories: Adolescence

I have more memories than if I were a thousand years old.
— Charles Baudelaire

Finally, in 1915, Hanna managed to return to Kraków, which by now was showing all the signs of having become a garrison town for the Austrian army, housing not only Austrian officers, but also regular soldiers in makeshift barracks. This was due in part to the town's good supply of ready-made buildings for billeting and many others which could be quickly converted into military hospitals or barracks. For several kilometres, all around the town, military barracks were hastily being constructed for the imperial Austrian army. It was during this time that the Austrian army built for its cavalry officers a series of red-brick barracks outside the small market town of Oświęcim, roughly twenty kilometres from Kraków. Twenty-five years later, these severe looking military buildings were to form the nucleus for the infamous Nazi concentration camp known to the rest of the world as Auschwitz.

In 1917, Hanna's parents decided to send her to a private convent school in Kraków run by the Ursuline Sisters of the Roman Union, which still provides education today. This was a well-known and well-run convent school for girls, with an excellent academic record, which prepared its students for the Austrian matriculation (i.e. high school) examination. At the time that Hanna attended the school, the majority of its teaching staff including the principal — Dr Karol Stach — were secular teachers. In time, however, these lay teachers were replaced by religious teaching sisters, as already in 1910, under the leadership of Mother Urszula Ledóchowska (1865-1939), the sisters had received special permission from the Church authorities to attend the Jagiellonian University, in order to obtain the necessary educational qualifications to be able to teach at the high school themselves. This demonstrates the forward-thinking nature of Mother Urszula. Her principal objective, however, was probably to facilitate keeping a closer control over the moral and spiritual development of the girls in their charge, rather than to enhance the intellectual development of the sisters.

At the time of the Great War, when Hanna was there, the school had over 300 pupils, which attests to its popularity. But by then, Mother Urszula had already left Austrian Galicia to help set up and run an academy for young girls in St Petersburg, in Imperial Russia. Mother Urszula, separated from her convent in Kraków by the Great War and later by the Russian Revolution of 1917 and the ensuing Russian civil war, went on to establish a new branch of Ursuline sisters. In 2003, this forward-thinking, dynamic woman — Mother Urszula Ledóchowska — was canonised in Rome, by Pope John Paul II. Hanna attended the school just after its charismatic headmistress, Saint Urszula, had left, but something of the ambiance left behind by Mother Urszula must have been felt by the students and staff. According to Hanna, however, some things did revert back to "the old ways", but, unfortunately for us, she does not elaborate on what these "old ways" may have been.

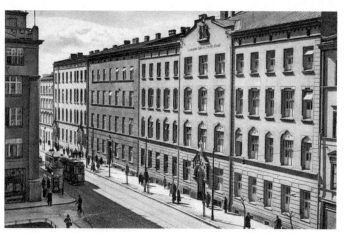

Ursuline Convent School, Kraków, 1930s

Meanwhile, attendance at this type of a school was for Hanna a completely new experience. First of all, the school was open to any girl whose family could afford to pay the fees and pass the entrance test. Secondly, just being at a school was a novel experience for Hanna, and the school's clear religious orientation was also something new for her. Although Hanna enjoyed the company of girls in the school and the friendships that resulted, not to mention the academic challenges, she was not particularly appreciative of the prevailing religious atmosphere which the sisters provided, such as the various para-liturgical services so prevalent in pre-Vatican II days, or obligatory participation in Sodality of Mary meetings and other devotional practices which were so common at that time.

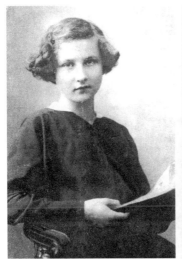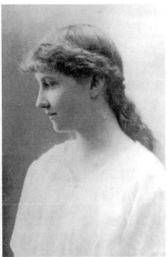

Hanna as a young student of the Ursuline Convent School and as an adolescent.

Over thirty years later, she wrote of the school that everything appeared to her to be new and even exotic. She noted, "The professors — what types! School-chums — what a wonderful collection of girls! A gradual introduction into the secrets of Polish literature, especially Old Slavonic literature. Our class was considered not only by us, but also by our teachers, to be first-rate, and differing from other classes by its specific character of social consciousness, a gift for organisation and patriotic spirit." Her estimation of the class seems to have been confirmed by other past pupils of the school and teachers; meanwhile, their recollection of Hanna from that time was that of an exceptionally gifted student and that the entire class was indeed unusually intellectually bright and social-minded.

Among her classmates and friends were the daughters of professors from the Jagiellonian University, so not only were the girls attending the same school, but their parents worked at the same university. Hanna's closest school-friend was Zofia Wajda, who was to share many years of close friendship with Hanna until her untimely death during the Second World War. Hanna wrote about her almost fifty years later, "I saw then and I see now her greatness, in every respect... in my [youthful] heart I used to call her 'Snow'. She deserves an ode, but I am incapable of writing it." Such gracious praise is rare and, in this context, where death had separated the two women for over thirty years, it is an unusual testament, saying as much about Hanna's own gracious personality as about the perceived goodness of her school-friend.

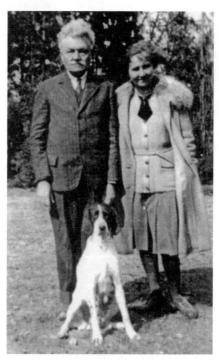

Hanna with her father.

The vast majority of students upon leaving the school went on to attend the Jagiellonian University (which unusually for educational institutions of higher learning at that time admitted women to full academic degrees), or other institutions of higher learning, such as medical schools, academies of fine arts or institutes of home economics. Hanna's closest friend, Zofia Wajda, chose to study medicine, while Hanna, upon completing her secondary education, could only think of one thing: how to structure her life so that she could work as a nurse.

At the same time as Hanna was finishing her basic education at the Ursuline Convent School in Kraków, the Great War was drawing to a close, and with its conclusion came the opportunity for Poland to demand its independence from the three occupying powers: Tsarist Russia, Prussia and the Austro-Hungarian Empire. Patriotic Kraków was buzzing with activity and talk of impending independence. On the morning of 11 November 1918, the newly-formed provisional Polish government handed over its interim powers to Marshall Józef Piłsudzki, who had arrived in Warsaw by train that very morning, having just been released twenty-four hours before, from a Prussian prisoner-of-war camp. The Second Polish Republic was formally declared. After almost a hundred and fifty years of non-sovereignty, Poland became a united and independent state once again. Hanna states in her memoirs, that as an adolescent she was an avid supporter of Marshall Piłsudzski's Polish Legions (battalions formed in 1914 in Kraków and fighting for Polish independence), much to the amazement and concern of her parents. This is not surprising, for at the time, these battalions did not always have the best of reputations. But young Hanna, who was staunchly patriotic, overlooked any negative aspects of the soldier's activities and only saw them as glorious liberators.

The English writer Monica Gardner, in a somewhat over-romanticised version of Polish history, concluded her book *A History of Poland*, with the accurate observation that "...we are mistaken if we believe that Poland owes her deliverance to the Great War. How was it that after more than a hundred years of pitiless persecution under the heel of three mighty conquerors there was any Polish nation left to be restored?"

For young Hanna, on the threshold of her adult life, this was an unforgettable moment, and a determining factor in her political orientation and her patriotic outlook. From now on Hanna knew she would be working for a free and independent Poland, and saw a future for herself in that autonomous country. She desired to work for change in what was, from now on to be an independent and self-governing country. Hanna was brought up by her parents to be a Polish patriot, to identify with *Polishness*, and the so-called *Polish Tradition*. This preparation in *Polishness* was now to be utilised to the full. For young people of Hanna's generation the work to be done in re-establishing one sovereign state from the remnants of the three parts that were Galicia, Prussian-occupied western Poland and the Russian-occupied central and eastern lands, was a gargantuan task. It is a tribute to the organisational skills, talents and tenacity of that generation of young people that so much was achieved by way of establishing a Polish state at all, in the short period between 1918 and 1939, before yet another war was to interrupt the political process of that precarious developing nation.

Hanna wanted to immediately throw herself into the work of rebuilding a free Poland, but before she could do anything, the war casualties both from the First World War and from the Polish-Bolshevik war who had been sent to the military hospitals of Kraków still needed to be attended to. With her friend Zofia Wajda she enrolled in a two-week Red Cross first aid course, organised by the American Red Cross, and she volunteered to work for the summer in an army hospital based at Kraków railway station.

Hanna recalls many funny stories from this time of her adolescent life, which she recounts with evident glee in her memoirs. When not attending to the wounded, together with Zofia she was sent by the Red Cross authorities to beg for money and alms from the good citizens of Kraków. The two girls thoroughly enjoyed themselves going around Kraków, knocking on people's doors and collecting donations of various sorts for the Red Cross. The girls were equally enthusiastic about working on the wards of the military hospital, and Hanna notes that the soldiers (most of whom were on the mend by this stage) hugely enjoyed their infectious humour and their youthful exuberance. But she also wrote that the hard work in the military hospital strongly influenced the future orientation of her career.

It was during this Red Cross course and her work with the wounded soldiers in Kraków that she met for the first time with the

American nurse educator of Polish parentage, Miss Stella Tylska, whom she was to encounter again several years later in Warsaw, in the newly opened Warsaw School of Nursing. However difficult and challenging Hanna may have found the Red Cross work, it convinced her more than ever that she wanted to be a nurse. Just how impressionable she was and the extent to which she was moved by what she heard and saw, can be judged by a comment she made in her autobiography written many decades later, '…to this day I can hear the screams of the young soldiers'.

The girls were working in the military hospital in the summer and autumn of 1920, while they were waiting to start their academic studies at the Jagiellonian University. Zofia had already been accepted to study medicine, and Hanna, in the absence of a school of nursing in Poland, chose to study Polish language and literature. No doubt she was influenced in her choice of subject by the prevailing humanistic atmosphere at home.

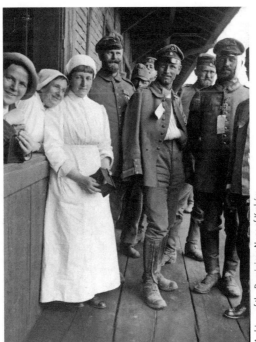

Archives of the Dominican Nuns of Kraków

Dressing Station at Kraków railway station, 1918

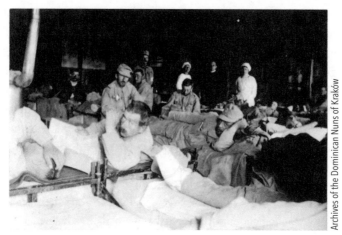

Archives of the Dominican Nuns of Kraków

Wounded soldiers at the Dressing Station (Kraków Railway Station)

CHAPTER 4

I Always Wanted to be a Nurse: Young Adulthood

'In my beginning is my end.'

— TS Eliot

The academic year 1920-21 commenced with a two-month delay because of the onset of the Polish-Bolshevik war. It was not until 2 December 1920 that Hanna Chrzanowska could finally register at the Department of Philosophy and Philology at Jagiellonian University. The prevailing scholarly atmosphere at home and easy access to books on philosophy and the humanities made this an obvious choice of study for the young woman, but she would have much preferred to have enrolled in a nursing school.

Many years later, she answered a question that many a sympathiser might be tempted to pose, and that is: why did she not choose a medical career if she was so intelligent and keen to alleviate suffering and wanted to work in a hospital? Certainly she had all the necessary intellectual gifts to undertake rigorous medical training and a family that would have been supportive of such a move. Hanna explains that she could easily have registered to study medicine with her friend Zofia, but it was not a career in medicine that appealed to her; she only wanted to be a nurse. She wrote in her memoirs, 'I did not want to study medicine. Never in my life have I regretted that I am not a physician. Instinctively I knew that medicine was one profession and nursing was something entirely different. I simply felt this distinction in the depth of my being, long before I could theoretically describe it. Also, not only was nursing something else, it was something higher. My mother always wanted me to undertake some form of social action.' For Hanna, nursing was always seen as a form of social action, an activity initially almost exclusively perceived by her as secular in nature, but which as time progressed, and her spirituality matured, was to become a practical and indeed an extraordinary example of Catholic Social Teaching — a truly Christian response to the call for a generosity of spirit, as elaborated upon and required of us in the evangelical account of the Sermon on the Mount and in the pages of the gospels.

The separation that inevitably occurred between the two friends as they pursued their separate careers was a great wrench for Hanna, and had she been less determined to be a nurse she might well have chosen to follow a career in medicine just to be with her friend. Hanna, however, wanted to follow a career in nursing, and enrolling at the Jagiellonian University to study the humanities was not a change of plan, rather it was simply a way to give herself more time to decide how best to go about becoming a nurse. In 1971, two years before her death, Hanna confirmed her life's choice of work when delivering a paper at a conference in Warsaw. She said, quoting Florence Nightingale, 'I dare to affirm that the happiest people, those most in love with their profession, most grateful for the gift of life, are those women who dedicate themselves to nursing.'

Because nursing schools did not exist in Poland at that time, a bold plan was needed, one which would involve traveling abroad to train as a nurse, just as her Aunt Zofia had done several years previously. But for the time being, Hanna chose to pursue a course of studies in the humanities, which seemed to her a safe option. Such studies would at least nourish her artistic tendencies, broaden her outlook on life and serve her well in any decisions about her future career. Hanna certainly did not see this move as a betrayal of her primary wish, rather as a stalling tactic that would, in the meantime, at least appeal to her artistic nature.

In the 1920s at the Jagiellonian University Department of Polish Language and Literature, Hanna came into contact with some of the greatest names in Polish studies, starting with her father. Not only did Hanna attend lectures in Polish Studies, but she also enrolled in classes on the history of art and of philology of Germanic and Romance languages. But as she noted, despite having a brilliant mind and being culturally prepared to benefit from these studies, she was neither particularly happy nor satisfied. So when, in the spring of 1921, Hanna was informed by her mother that a professional nursing school was to be established in Warsaw called the Warsaw School of Nursing (*Warszawska Szkoła Pielęgniarska*), she was ecstatic. The school was founded and to be operated through the combined efforts of the American Red Cross, the Rockefeller Foundation, several private benefactors including her aunt, Zofia Szlenkier, and the world-famous diplomat-pianist and philanthropist — Ignacy Paderewski (1860-1941).

The first nurse-tutors at the school were all American women, and some were of Polish descent, such as Miss Aleksandra Zarzycka, Miss Julia Wolska and Miss Stella Tylska. Hanna had already come into contact with some of them in Kraków at the end of the First World War, while attending the Red Cross training course.

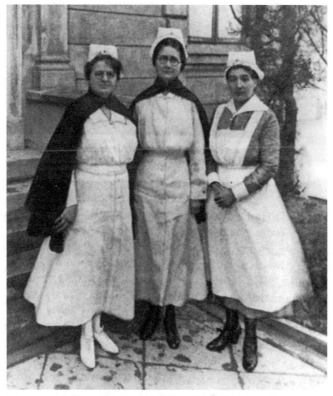

American Red Cross Nurses with Miss Helen Bridge in the centre and Stella Tylska on the left. Kraków during World War I.

Miss Helen Bridge, who despite her title had married twice, was appointed by the American Red Cross to be the first Nursing Director. She had no Polish connections prior to her arrival in Poland, but she had worked in several other countries, setting up nurse training schools for the International Red Cross, supported by the Rockefeller Foundation. Immediately prior to working in Poland however, she had been Director of the Illinois Nurse Training School in the USA, having returned from a tour of duty with the American Red Cross setting up nursing schools in Mongolia and Siberia. Speaking no Polish when she first arrived in Poland, all her initial dealings with the students and Polish staff were conducted through an interpreter, until she learnt sufficient Polish to manage on her own.

Hanna immediately decided to transfer from Polish studies at the Jagiellonian University to the Warsaw School of Nursing (WSN), in pursuit of a nursing career. Hanna's father agreed to his daughter's change of studies, but there were some in Kraków who raised protesting voices to the effect that social standards must indeed be falling if Professor Chrzanowski allowed his daughter to go to a *nursing* school.

In order to prepare herself for the October intake of nursing students, Hanna arranged to spend the intervening six months working as a volunteer at a clinic for the poor in Kraków. The clinic was run by the Association of Lady Almoners (*Towarzystwo Panien Ekonomek*). They were a charitable, mainly fund-raising organisation, working under the leadership and direction of the Daughters of Charity of St Vincent de Paul and Miss Maria Epstein (1875-1947), a rich, highly-talented and devout woman who was to profoundly affect Hanna and who accompanied Hanna's nursing career over the next decades. In her memoirs Hanna recounts their first meeting, when Maria received her most warmly. Hanna recalls that in Maria's office was a sideboard full of exquisite Danish porcelain. She continues in her memoirs that it is with great joy that she will be coming back to writing about Miss Maria Epstein (whom she liked and appreciated a lot) in her 'autobiography'.

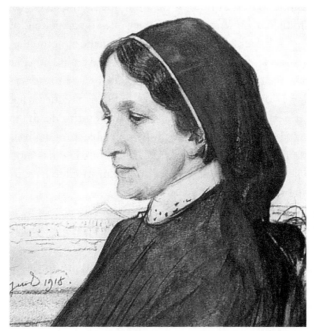

Servant of God Maria Epstein as a Lady Almoner. In 2004 her
canonisation cause was formally opened in the chapel of the cloistered
Dominican nuns of Kraków. Painting by L. Wyczółkowski.

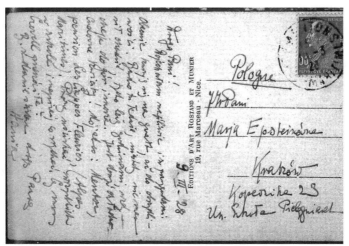

Postcard Hanna sent to Maria Epstein from Menton, in 1928.

Hanna was given various responsibilities at the clinic, which the Association ran on Warszawska Street, including looking after the association's ledger and sorting out their financial accounts. Hanna admits that she could not do this last job, and frankly did not want to. This is one of the few instances where Hanna admits that she was beaten and sufficiently stubborn not to fulfil her assigned responsibilities. Besides, as she said, she really did not want to do the job. One sees Hanna here, possibly at her most vulnerable, running back to the nest to find support from her parents. Apparently Hanna's mother saw the predicament coming and was not at all surprised to have to step in and help her daughter out.

The opening of the Warsaw School of Nursing came about at the very best moment for Hanna, and in March 1922 she was accepted into the second intake of students with 21 other like-minded women. In this manner she finally embarked on her long dreamed-of nursing career. The WSN had been open just six months when Hanna started her training, and it still had the atmosphere of a pioneering establishment trying to iron out unexpected glitches. The academic level of the school, however, was never in question. It followed a two-year programme, the accepted length of training in the USA and in Britain at that time, and was open to any young woman who had successfully gained her matriculation certificate (high school diploma) and was considered to be of worthy character. The entrance qualifications required of students applying to the school of nursing in Warsaw, during those early years, were the same as those required for acceptance to university studies or teacher training. This would suggest that those first Polish nursing students possessed academic qualifications in excess of requirements in many comparable schools of nursing elsewhere in Europe at that time. But it was one of the aims of the Rockefeller Foundation that the school was to educate those first nursing students in such a way that the new nurses would be ready to become the nurse educators and leaders of the future, an expectation which might help explain to some extent the rigorous entrance requirements.

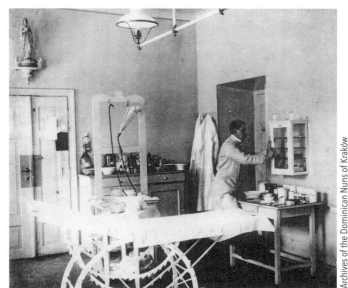

Archives of the Dominican Nuns of Kraków

Dispensary of the Lady Almoners where Hanna worked for
Maria Epstein.

Students paid a fee to attend, and all the nursing students had to reside in the nurses' home, where they slept several to a room, dormitory style. Conditions were Spartan, and food was scarce and, according to Hanna, also extremely unappetising. On the first day they were given pickled herrings in batter for supper, a dish which the young women found very difficult to eat; but Hanna who even as a child felt that in order to train her will-power she should occasionally eat spoonfuls of salt mixed with sugar, devoured an entire plate of the dubious fish meal, to the amazement of everyone at the table. The discipline at the school was so rigorous that many years later Hanna would comment on the rigid rules governing the lives of the young women. Some of these hardships were due no doubt to the nature of nursing schools at that time, and some to the consequences of economic hardship prevailing in the country during those grim depression years, which affected the whole of Europe, including Poland — as much as the USA.

Many of the women entering the WSN were older than subsequent candidates; Hanna herself was twenty. The age-range in her nursing set was from 18 to 46. The difficult conditions in the school must have been felt quite keenly by these mature women who had seen war, had often managed their own affairs, and had become accustomed to making independent decisions. Hanna commented at some length on the almost pointless hardships which the school imposed on the young nursing students. She noted that she obeyed the rules not so much out of fear as out of a sense of duty. However, if she did break some rules, it was only 'the more absurd ones'.

Hanna recounts a hilarious incident in her memoirs when together with her cousin Fijka, who was also studying nursing at the WSN, the two women managed to creep into the demonstration room in the school one evening, and proceeded to practise giving bed-baths, to each other — ending up with water spilt all over the floor and wet sheets on the demonstration beds... Hanna does not say what reprimand was given to them, but the tutors at the time, were apparently not as amused as Hanna seems to have been, many decades later, when joyfully recalling the incident. In the time-honoured fashion of nurses recounting their Preliminary Training School (PTS) days, Hanna notes that she needed six safety pins (and an assortment of buttons and hooks) to fix her starched apron and uniform. She also recalls how during her first meal in the school dining-room, the students from the first intake regaled the new (second intake) students with horrific stories of blood and gore that was awaiting them on the wards.

It is not clear why, but of the 21 students who started the course, only 14 managed to complete it. Hanna observed that students were ordered to leave on the slightest pretext, and she characteristically added, 'and it's not clear that it was the best girls who survived the course to the end'. In keeping with English and American nursing programmes at that time, almost 80 percent of the training was taken up with practical sessions on hospital wards and if one was fortunate, a tiny amount of exposure to practice in the community. Among the hospitals to which the students were sent for practical sessions was the Children's Hospital of Charles and Mary, the very hospital founded by Hanna's aunt and where Hanna herself had been an in-patient as a child. Hanna had nothing but praise for the approach of her nurse tutors towards patients and the dignity of their nursing work and one can see the effects of their exemplary professionalism on the passionate approach of Hanna towards her own patient care, several decades later.

In spite of the hardships imposed on the students, Hanna

managed to bring to her fellow nursing students moments of amuse-
ment and joy. As in her time at the Ursuline convent school in Kraków,
her sense of humour and fun became legendary. Her friends at the
nursing school quickly recognised her ability to introduce cheer even
into the bleakest of circumstances. It was her sheer joy in life and
contagious laughter that her peers would, years later, remember most
vividly. As Hanna herself noted, 'my antics in no way prevented me
from working,' and with her close friends she got up to all sorts of
adventures.

At the school, much emphasis was put on tidiness and clean-
liness. Hanna, who for most of her life found it difficult to keep her
immediate environment tidy, and was known even as a mature nurse-
teacher to have a hard time keeping her records and work in order,
relates how one day at nursing school she returned from her duty on
the wards to find an envelope addressed to herself with a note from
Miss Helen Bridge: 'Dear Miss Chrzanowska, are there any reasons
why you should be less tidy in your dormitory cupboard than on the
wards? Yours Sincerely, Helen L. Bridge.' Eventually, after many years,
Hanna's tidiness did improve — but it was not easy

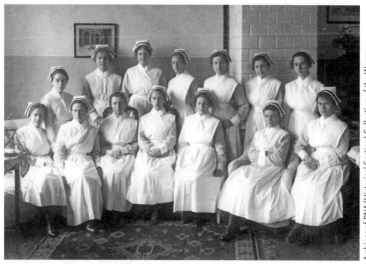

Archives of PNA (Historical Section) Collection of the Warsaw
School of Nursing

Hanna with her graduating class from the Warsaw School of Nursing.
Hanna is standing first from the left in the back row.

On 30 June 1924, Hanna completed her studies at the WSN, and she left that very evening on the late train, returning straight to Kraków. As she later wrote, she did not intend to be at the school so much as an hour longer than was absolutely necessary. Hanna respected the education she received at the school but found its rules crippling and confining. Like students the world over, she wanted to start enjoying her freedom as soon as possible. That the education she received at the school was considered excellent, even by non-nursing standards, was made evident in 1938, when graduates of the school, with a few other selected professions, were allowed to vote for the Polish Upper Chamber — the Senate. At that time, only one per cent of the Polish population had the right to vote for the upper chamber, and among that one per cent were qualified nurses.

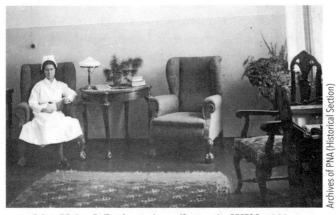

Miss Helen L Bridge in her office in the WSN, 1920s.

Archives of PNA (Historical Section)

A few months before she completed her studies however, Hanna was invited to the office of the Directress, Helen Bridge. She asked Hanna if she would like to consider going to Paris for several months to study community nursing care. The authorities at the Rockefeller Foundation had chosen Hanna and her nursing school friend Zofia Wasilewska to continue their nursing studies abroad with the intention that upon their return to Poland they would help set up further nursing courses, specifically in the area of public health and community nursing. Such scholarships were aimed at improving nurse training and educating future nurse leaders and teachers. It was a novel undertaking by the Rockefeller Foundation, and one that proved to be far-sighted, especially in the Polish context. Hanna's exposure to community and child health nursing in France was to totally change her hitherto hospital-based impression of nursing-care and it determined the future orientation of her nursing career.

Going to Paris would ultimately lead to Hanna setting up a professional community nursing programme in Kraków. Additionally, Helen Bridge wanted Hanna to help re-establish a school of nursing in Kraków, along modern professional lines, like the new Warsaw School, and to be responsible for its community nursing department. Their knowledge of French, their outgoing personalities and pleasant social manners must have also played a part in the decision to send the pair to France. Hanna was so delighted at the proposition that several years later, Miss Bridge who was visiting Poland at the time commented that, 'Hanna was dancing on the edge of her chair at the proposal'.

Although Hanna and her companion were ready to travel to France immediately, there was a considerable delay in finalising the necessary paperwork and organising the visas and passports. While they waited for these formalities to be completed, Hanna decided to spend the intervening academic year 1924/25 continuing her Polish studies, which had been interrupted three years earlier, at the Jagiellonian University. This love of the humanities and literature was to persist throughout Hanna's life and regardless of how busy her professional nursing life would become, she always found the time to go to the theatre or art gallery, attend a concert or read a good book.

She did not arrive in Paris, therefore, until 6 January 1925, on the feast of the Epiphany. But as Hanna noted in her memoirs, the feast held little significance for her at that time. It was only in retrospect, that Hanna saw her stay in Paris as the beginning of something far more wonderful and fulfilling than simply an exciting study-visit, and that her arrival in Paris on 6 January was an interesting spiritual pointer to her future faith. As she said years later, with candid honesty, she was not aware at the time of the religious significance of many of the dates in the Christian calendar. More amazingly, she was not even overly concerned with the professional nature of her studies in Paris. She was engrossed in the reality of just being *in* Paris — the fulfilment of her young life's dream. For once, at least initially, nursing considerations took second place.

The young women marvelled like excited children at the luxurious fittings in their sleeper compartment, which had been booked for them from Warsaw to Paris. The pair arrived at Gare du Nord railway station in Paris, and were immediately taken by taxi to the northern suburbs of the city — to the nurses' home of the Children's Hospital on Rue Desonettes. The young women were so giggly and enthusiastic during this last leg of the journey that Hanna commented years later in her memoires that it is surprising the taxi-driver did not take them straight to the local psychiatric hospital instead!

The director of the school of nursing, Mlle. Marguerite Grenier (who was also *Surveillante générale de l'école d'infirmières de l'Assistance publique de Paris* – a nursing school inspector) was a founding member of the French Nursing Association. She worked closely with Mme. Léonie Chaptal — president of the French association and subsequently president of the International Council of Nurses from 1929-1933. Léonie Chaptal was a devout Catholic, and was also a founding member of the International Association of Catholic Nurses. It was Mme Chaptal who helped to organise the first general meeting of the Catholic nurses association in 1934 in Lourdes. Several years later a few of Hanna's close friends and colleagues were to attend that international meeting and would write up their impressions for the Polish Nurse's journal — of which Hanna was to become the editor-in-chief. But all that activity lay ahead of Hanna; in 1925 she was still a young, inexperienced, newly qualified nurse. She did comment however in her memoirs that she was very fond of Mlle Grenier, whom she found to be wise and caring.

Meanwhile, these energetic, well-educated, powerful French women, who were the leaders of the newly founded nursing profession in France, cooperated closely with the International Red Cross and the Rockefeller Foundation and were now intent on passing on their nursing expertise and knowledge to the next generation of young women. Sadly, the school and paediatric hospital that Hanna and her friend attended on Rue Desonettes no longer exists, having been bulldozed to make way for the building of the Paris orbital highway, the so-called Périphérique.

The daily routine in the French school was not dissimilar from what the young women had grown to accept in Warsaw, but there were some local differences — mostly to do with food — both its quantity and quality. Hanna observed years later that the two Polish women arrived at the school of nursing on the feast of Epiphany, at exactly the right time for supper, and that it was a pleasant surprise to observe the French students studiously examining the piece of cake on their plates, apparently intently looking for a tiny porcelain figurine which had been put into the cake by the cook. Once the little figurine was found, the lucky person was declared King for the rest of the day, amid much laughter and banter. Similar Epiphany customs exist to this day in many Catholic countries of Europe, including Poland.

While Hanna studied and observed the organisation of community and paediatric care in Paris, she also threw herself with great enthusiasm into getting to know the city, its museums, art galleries, ancient monuments and buildings. Just how well she got to know the city is apparent from her first semi-autobiographical novel, *Niebieski Klucz* (The Key to Heaven), where the entire action takes place in Paris, mostly on the Left Bank of the River Seine. From that short book one can create an interesting walk around Hanna's Paris, one which reflects her time there studying community nursing and exploring the riches of that fascinating city.

She regularly attended concerts at the old Conservatory and would discuss musical matters at some length with Mlle Marguerite Greiner, the director of the School of Nursing, who encouraged the two Polish women to attend as many concerts as they could. According to Hanna, Mlle Greiner enjoyed listening to Beethoven and considered the opening of his Fifth Symphony to be some of his finest music, often commenting, *'Elle est si douce'*, [It is so sweet.] The younger but more musically aware Hanna, did not dare to contradict her, so strongly had been the idea of subordination inculcated into the nursing students in Warsaw. But, characteristically, Hanna added in her autobiographical notes, 'Besides, we were fond of her and had great respect for her.' It is impossible to say to what extent Mlle Greiner influenced Hanna's subsequent taste in music, but as a mature woman, Hanna was also known to prefer Beethoven to other classical composers.

Hanna would write about this time, not surprisingly, in glowing terms: her enthusiasm for her Parisian interlude is very obvious to the reader of her memoirs. At some point Hanna visited and worked in other centres in France, including Lyon, Nancy and Strasbourg. A few photographs survive of Hanna in Strasbourg, but she does not elaborate on these other nursing placements in her memoirs.

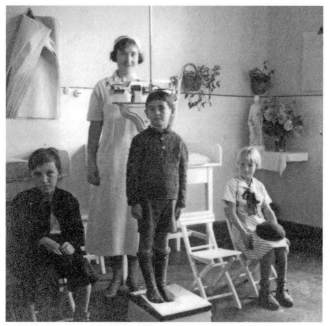

Hanna weighing children

We know from a letter of confirmation sent in 1999 from the Rockefeller Foundation in New York to the Catholic Nurses Association in Kraków that Hanna was sent (as were most other recipients of Rockefeller scholarships) to these other centres of nursing excellence in France apart from Paris, centres which were deemed at the time to illustrate the best in public health nursing and community care.

CHAPTER 5

Responsibility For My Profession:
A Spectacular Nursing Career

*Nursing became a service requiring high qualifications, with a
sense of engagement and social responsibility.*
— S. Poznańska

On 10 December 1925, after several years of effort, a new modern
secular nursing school was finally re-established in Kraków. A school
had previously existed for a short while, but it was run along religious
lines, by Maria Epstein and The Association of Lady Almoners, and
it had to close in 1921 after functioning for only ten years, due to lack
of funds. The new modern school was conducted along the lines of the
school in Warsaw, and also benefited from the financial backing of The
Rockefeller Foundation. Maria Epstein was nominated to be its first
Directress, thus providing the necessary continuity and expertise. That
same year, Hanna returned to Kraków, and in accordance with her
agreement with The Rockefeller Foundation, she started working with
Maria Epstein to establish the Kraków School of Nursing.

Maria Epstein was a deeply religious woman, and so the new
nursing school, much like the previous school, was steeped in religious
tradition. It had a chapel, which the students attended on Sundays
and major feasts; and they were given sessions on moral and spiritual
development, while yearly retreats were conducted by some of the best
known spiritual directors in Kraków. Hanna was unimpressed by this
obvious "show" of religiosity, as she commented to friends at the time.
She saw no need to bring religious education, and especially retreats,
into the nursing school environment or curriculum.

Cardinal Adam Sapieha (1867-1951) Archbishop of Kraków
at the time and a significant personality in the Polish and universal

Church, was a personal friend, confessor and supporter of Maria Epstein and her works. He was a frequent visitor to the school. But after only five years at the new school, Maria Epstein resigned as its director and in 1930 entered the enclosed monastery of Dominican nuns on Mikołajska Street, in Kraków. Much later, in 2008, the Dominican nuns in Kraków instigated her canonisation process – she is now known as Servant of God Sister Magdalena, OP. It is hoped that her enormous contribution to nursing, the church and the town of Kraków will soon become more widely known. It may well be that the people of Kraków will now be praying to Blessed Hanna for the speedy canonisation of her one-time mentor, Sister Maria Magdalena Epstein.

As the unfolding story of Hanna's life will show, it is amazing how many holy and influential people knew each other and worked together for the common good in Poland, firstly in those heady inter-war years and then later during the Communist period — all drawn to each other like bees drawn to a celestial honey-pot. It was a veritable communion of saints.

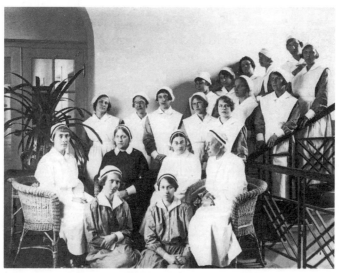

Hanna as a young nurse teacher – sitting on the ground directly below Maria Epstein (in black) the director of the Kraków School of Nursing.

The new nursing school was incorporated into the Medical Academy of the Jagiellonian University, giving it university status, a rarity for nursing schools in those days. It was regarded as a totally autonomous institution within the academy, in control of its own standards and programme of studies. Because the School was a department of the University, it benefited from the university lecture theatres, laboratories, and professorial input for specialist lectures. For clinical and practical experience, the students had access to the consultants' wards at the University Medical Hospitals on Kopernika Street.

Hanna was to be associated with this school through all of its phases, off and on, for the rest of her life. She worked there as an instructor of community nursing and nursing care of the newborn, from 1 February 1926 to May 1929. At that time in Poland, most births took place at home, and so her two areas of teaching and clinical concerns were somewhat related. Meanwhile, on 26 April 1926, she sat her state examinations to qualify as a *registered* nurse, in accordance with the requirements of the Ministry of Health. In June of that year, upon receiving her state certificate with a final grade of *excellent*, Hanna not only became a graduate of the prestigious WSN but also formally became recognised by the Polish State as a registered professional nurse. Her childhood dream of becoming a nurse had come true.

Shortly after she started to work at the school in Kraków, she was sent abroad once again for a few months, on another Rockefeller stipend, but this time to Belgium to look at, and acquaint herself with, the role and training of school nurses. The newly established Polish Ministry of Health wanted to provide the best, most affordable, universal, and holistic care for its citizens, starting with antenatal provision, community-based health centres, and resources for school-age children. Hanna's educational trip to Belgium was necessary for the implementation of Poland's vision of comprehensive community healthcare, and it was in keeping with Hanna's own emerging professional interests. Emphasis on the significance of public health and provision for community health care needs was also one of the long-term strategies of both the Red Cross and the Rockefeller Foundation; this also coincided with the larger healthcare and social plans of the main philanthropic foundations operating in central Europe at that time.

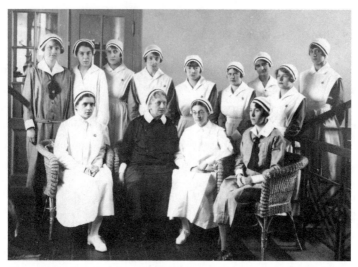

Hanna (standing first from the left) as a young instructor of community nursing in Kraków. Maria Epstein (in black) is in the centre.

In 1927, the Rockefeller Foundation donated $100,000 (representing a sixth of the costs) towards the long awaited construction of a purpose-built building in which to permanently house the Warsaw School of Nursing. The building was officially opened on 11 May 1930 in the presence of government officials, municipal dignitaries and the President's wife, Mrs. Mościcka — as well as Hanna's Aunt Zofia Szlenkier, who was Directress of the School of Nursing at that time. She became the first directress of the school after Helen Bridge returned to USA. However, it is not known for certain whether Hanna or indeed any of that first intake of pioneering nursing students were also present at the ceremony.

Throughout the 1930's, the Rockefeller Foundation not only supported individual healthcare professionals enabling them to specialise and to broaden their clinical expertise, but it also contributed large sums of money in the USA and around the world towards building clinics, hospitals and schools of nursing and medicine. Hanna was well aware of the role that the Rockefeller Foundation played in promoting healthcare issues in Poland, and she wrote an article in 1937 for the Polish nursing journal *Pielęgniarka Polska* about the activities of the foundation in Poland.

Upon returning to Poland from Belgium, she took over the responsibility for the provision of school nursing at two primary schools in Kraków, St Nicholas' and St Anne's, where her nursing students also had their community placements. During this time, Hanna also set up a drop-in advisory centre for pregnant women, attached to the Medical Academy's antenatal clinic. It was run solely by nurses, and this too became a community placement for her students. Increasingly, though wanting to be a hospital-based nurse, Hanna found herself focusing on the nursing needs of patients in the community. In time she grew not only to adopt this area of work as her own, but to identify herself totally with this form of nursing service.

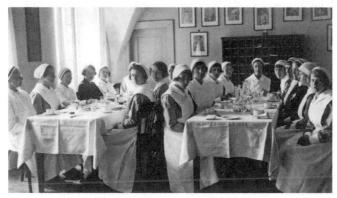

Dining room in the Kraków School of Nursing. Hanna is sitting 2nd from the right on the table by the window.

Miss Epstein scrupulously noted, however, in her yearly staff evaluation reports, that Hanna had been absent from work for eight weeks due to ill health. Indeed, Hanna's bad health necessitated her resignation from the school in May 1929 and she went to a sanatorium in Zakopane and in Davos, Switzerland, for further treatment. In Davos, Hanna wrote the first of her three semi-autobiographical novels under the title, *Niebieski Klucz* (The Key to Heaven), while the actual experience of being in the Davos sanatorium was the inspiration for her last book *Płonący Śnieg* (Blazing Snow) which was written during the war and is still in manuscript form. It was never published. Although Hanna no longer taught at the school, she continued to busy herself with professional nursing matters.

Meanwhile, back in 1924, with the inspiration and support of Miss Helen Bridge, the newly qualified Polish registered nurses sought to establish their own professional nursing association. From its inception Hanna was an active member of the *Polskie Stowarzyszenie Pielęgniarek Zawodowych* (PSPZ) – The Polish Association of Professional Nurses. It was formally and legally established in Poland in 1925 and was officially accepted into the International Council of Nurses (ICN) in 1926. The first General Meeting of the National Council of Polish Professional Nurses was held in Warsaw in October 1926.

Hanna was to become an exemplary member of the association, working at national level in Warsaw with the Executive Council and also at regional and local level in Kraków. At the third Annual General Meeting of the Association in 1928, the Executive Council voted to establish a Polish professional nursing journal, and the first issue of *Pielęgniarka Polska* (Polish Nurse) appeared on the first of July 1929. Hanna was associated with the journal from the very beginning. Initially, she was co-editor with Jadwiga Suffczyńska, a close friend and colleague, and from June 1931 she became its Editor-in-chief. That Hanna would find much satisfaction from this work and be an exceptionally gifted editor is not surprising as she had proven artistic and writing talents and, in the tradition of her father, a well-formed literary style.

From 1932, the journal's offices were located on the fifth floor of the new building of the WSN in the centre of the city, at 78 Koszykowa Street. Beginning in 1933, her close friend from nursing school days, Maria Starowieyska, helped with the administrative side of the publication. Hanna additionally recruited some of the best names in Polish nursing to join the journal's editorial board, such as her colleague from the WSN, Aleksandra Dąmbska. Aleksandra would continue her friendship and co-operation with Hanna right up to Hanna's death in 1973. Shortly after becoming Editor-in-chief of the journal, Hanna moved her living quarters to the same floor as the journal's office. This move was probably the result of her being offered the position of vice-principal of the WSN and, therefore, may have reflected her desire to be closer to both the school *and* the editorial offices of the journal.

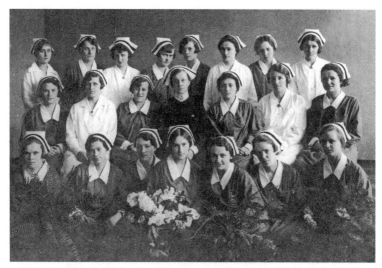

Warsaw School of Nursing, Hanna as a young nurse teacher – standing at the back, first in the last row from the left. Zofia Szlenkier in black in the centre.

Because of Hanna's strong interest in community nursing, from the first issue of the journal there was a strong emphasis on community nursing care, which was somewhat unusual among professional nursing journals of this period. Among the many topics Hanna wrote about were nursing and social problems associated with alcoholism and the care of patients with tuberculosis, organisational issues concerned with running nursing schools and proposals on how to establish nursing structures and hierarchies in hospitals — all reflecting current concerns in Poland and in Europe at that time.

Her friend Aleksandra, who was also a community nurse working in the eastern border town of Lwów (now Lvív, the capital of Western Ukraine), also contributed articles on community issues. Many of the articles on TB prevention and control (an enormous health problem at the time), were from Aleksandra Dąmbska's pen or written and published by Aleksandra's colleagues at her insistence and with her encouragement. The two friends ensured that in the journal, community nursing care had a high profile.

In 1931, at the request of the Department of Health of the City of Warsaw, Hanna included in the journal a questionnaire on various aspects of nursing in community healthcare centres. This was but one example of the role that she saw the journal fulfilling and to which she gladly lent a hand. All the issues contained nursing research reports, and often distinguished physicians and surgeons would contribute articles. From 1937, Hanna wrote a series of articles on nursing care based on the lecture notes of her mentor and senior colleague from the Kraków School of Nursing, Teresa Kulczyńska. In 1938, this series of articles was compiled and eventually published in book form and became an immediate nursing best-seller and a very popular textbook which saw many editions and reprints; interestingly, one reprint was issued for the benefit of Polish army nurses stationed in Scotland during the Second World War.

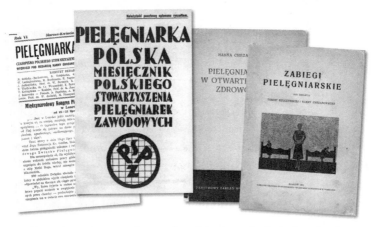

Hanna's textbooks and examples of the journal which she edited.

Hanna also brought to the journal an international dimension. Not only did she read and scan foreign press and overseas professional nursing and medical literature herself, but she also translated the more significant articles and items of information in order to include them in the Polish journal. From the beginning of her editorship, there appeared a regular column with nursing and medical news from around the world. After two years of work at the Warsaw School, ill health forced her to resign from her post as Assistant Director, and she left to seek rest and convalescent care in the Tatra Mountains.

In spite of leaving Warsaw, she continued as editor of the journal until 1939, and still took an active part in running the Nursing

Association. In 1939, with the onset of war with Germany imminent, she put an appeal in the journal for nurses to start collecting money to help finance a "hospital plane". The idea of the plane was inspired by reports from nurses who had worked in hospital trains and on hospital ships and barges during the First World War. The early outbreak of hostilities prevented the realisation of this project, but nurses did send money to the journal office, and interest in the project was high.

One of the notable public activities of the fledgling Nursing Association was advising and taking part in drafting legislation concerning nursing practice. The formal establishment of the nursing profession by the Polish legislature and Ministry of Health in 1935, with the participation of the nursing profession, was no small feat. At the Fifth Annual General Meeting of the Polish Nursing Association an item of business was covered concerning the drafting of a Nursing Bill and submitting it to the Ministry of the Interior for consideration. The prevailing atmosphere among the various healthcare professionals, lawyers and politicians seems to have been one of mutual respect and a genuine collaborative spirit in the interest of public health. The calibre of nurses working on the Nursing Bill must have had some effect on the tone and nature of the proceedings.

Hanna's strong personality was of immense significance. On 21 February 1935, the nursing profession was formally recognised by the Polish State, and few were as satisfied and proud of their input into the process of official recognition as Hanna and members of the Nursing Association itself. This 1935 nursing legislation, with only minor amendments, was to remain in force throughout the post-war years until the acceptance in 1997 by the post-Communist Polish Sejm and Senate (Combined Houses of the Polish Legislature) of a new Nursing Bill. The scope of the 1935 legislation was broad and covered not only predictable areas such as a definition of the nature of nursing and nursing practice and stating levels of competency and education, but also penal regulations and how the nursing body was to be structured, supervised and administered.

The Polish Government of 1935 had such a high regard for Hanna and her contribution to public health and nursing affairs that she received a governmental citation and medal in recognition of her hard work and her input into preparing the nursing legislation.

Likewise, in 1936 the profession itself, recognising her unique administrative and managerial talents and her dedication to the nursing profession, elected her as vice-president of its professional association, a position which Hanna held until the outbreak of the Second World War, when the association was closed down by the German authorities.

Hanna Chrzanowska was not only a dedicated nurse. It would be a huge injustice to her many gifts to state that she was simply 'wedded' to nursing. Although she always defined herself as a nurse, and was immensely proud to be one, she was a woman of many interests and talents. Although Hanna saw herself primarily as a professional woman, she was also committed to her family and concerned with the political and social affairs of the emerging Polish State; additionally, she had far-ranging interests in the humanities — reflected in her love of literature, theatre and music. Finally, she had a talent for creative writing. All her life she was known to enjoy 'the fine arts' and actively contributed to them, particularly through her novels, her poetry and other forms of writing.

CHAPTER 6

Painting with Words: A Talent for Writing

I can shake off everything as I write; my sorrows disappear, my courage is reborn.

— Anne Frank

Hanna wrote all her life, from early adolescence in high school, to shortly before her death — poems, short stories, novels, spoof doggerels in the style of limericks and illustrated cartoons with amusing comments. She also kept up a prolific correspondence with friends, colleagues and members of her extended family.

In 1934, her first novel *Klucz Niebieski* (The Key to Heaven) was published and in 1938, *Krzyż na Piasku* (A Cross in the Sand). Together with her last novel, *Płonący Śnieg* (Blazing Snow), they are to some extent autobiographical. Her *Memoirs*, were written in the late 1950's at the request of her parish nursing colleagues and for the younger generation of post-war nurses, and this combined literary legacy constitutes a substantial volume of writing. She had a lively and immediate style and a characteristic quality to her prose which makes the reading of her works quite thought-provoking. She had a masterly command of the Polish language — her prose being lyrical, sometimes to the point of being exuberant. But that was the accepted writing style at the time.

Hanna's *Memoirs* are probably her most engaging work. They are as readable today as when they were written and are probably of the most immediate interest to contemporary nursing and Catholic readerships. They are being currently edited and published in Kraków to coincide with Hanna's beatification. But her quasi-autobiographical novels, especially *The Key to Heaven* and *Blazing Snow*, also reveal her sensitivities, preoccupations and emerging interest in religion and, therefore, give us another glimpse into her spiritual development.

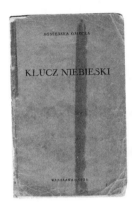
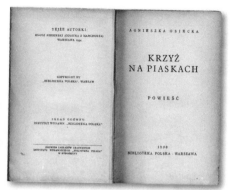

Two of Hanna's published semi-autobiographical novels.

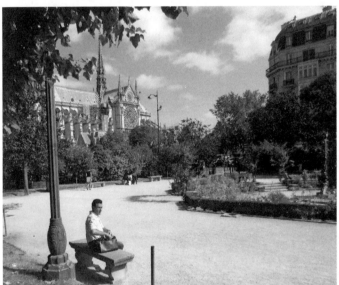

Hanna places the action of her book *Klucz Niebieski* – The Key to
Heaven, in the shadows of Notre Dame Cathedral and within the
Church of Notre Dame des Victoires.

Of more lasting literary interest, however, are her poems and
short stories. Hanna's niece, Dr Danuta Chrzanowska, recalls that as
a child she loved to go for walks with her Auntie Hanna, because
her aunt used to tell such wonderful stories. One involved the fate
of a fairy princess and her evil-minded chambermaid. This quixotic

and enchanting tale, recalled by Dr Chrzanowska but not surviving in written form, leads one to suspect that we will never know the true extent of Hanna's creative talent. Since most of her poetry and shorter artistic creations were never published, and most have not survived the turbulent war years, the true extent of her writing talent can never be adequately appraised.

Nonetheless, it seems to have been a rich talent and one which, unfortunately, was never taken seriously enough by Hanna herself. She saw it solely as a mechanism through which to amuse relatives and friends and through which she could put her thoughts and reflections down on paper — but mostly for her own personal relaxation or meditation. While Hanna's family and friends knew that she was a gifted composer of doggerels and lyrics, it would appear that they made no particular effort to preserve Hanna's more serious poems. On one occasion Hanna composed an ode, several pages long, for the wedding of a cousin. She did this while on a three-hour train journey from Kraków to Warsaw, on the way to the wedding ceremony.

Whenever Hanna's smaller works and poems were published in journals or newspapers, they were, like her novels, printed under the pseudonym *Agnieszka Osiecka*. She began to write as a schoolgirl, and many of her early poems appeared in the pre-war journal *Myśl Narodowa*. Her poem *A Christmas Carol*, probably written in the 1960's but only found among Hanna's papers after her death, is already becoming a favourite among Polish poetry-lovers. It is not a sentimental Nativity poem of the Victorian Christmas genre; rather it focuses on the natural womanly concerns expressed so eloquently nowadays by female poets. Hanna's poem articulates the worries of a concerned midwife, with all the urgency and love proper to her profession. It reflects the involvement of a caring nurse but is delivered in the gentle language of a poetic, insightful and compassionate woman.

Hanna's poems and her novels were concerned with issues which reflected her womanly, and increasingly, her religious interests. They are mirrors, which beautifully reflect her psyche and her moral development, and they are of major significance in assessing her spiritual development, her wisdom and sanctity. Sadly, it will never be known whether her papers and diaries, which were mostly destroyed immediately after her death, also contained poems or spiritual reflections.

During the last few years leading up to the Second World War, Hanna began to reflect on moral and spiritual issues. At this point she was already a mature woman, with substantial life experience behind her and with much expertise to share. She was in her mid-thirties but, characteristically, always open to new ideas, influences and possibilities. Under the influence of her colleagues and friends, whom she greatly admired and respected, she started to consider issues concerning her own development, spirituality and commitment to her Catholic faith.

A major contributing factor towards Hanna's readiness to start reflecting on matters of religion and spirituality was her ongoing professional relationship and close friendship with Maria Starowieyska, her friend from the WSN and more recently co-worker on the editorial board of the journal, *Pielęgniarka Polska*. Maria was a committed Christian, and it was her friendship which led Hanna to re-evaluate her dormant cradle-Catholic faith. Hanna the apathetic Catholic was slowly returning to the Church through Maria's gentle charm. That Maria Starowieyska was interested in a living faith which permeated her whole life and professional activities can be judged by the articles she wrote, some of them together with Hanna for *Pielęgniarka Polska*. One topic on which she wrote was the work of *The Catholic International Association of Professional Nurses*. Today this Association is known as The International Catholic Committee of Nurses and Medico-Social Assistants or *CICIAMS*. In 1933, Maria wrote a report for the journal from the international gathering of Catholic nurses in Lourdes, which she had just attended.

Hanna herself started to write articles for the journal which were Catholic, or hagiographic or spiritual in nature; for example about leprosy and Fr Damian, (now Saint Damian of Molokai), or about Fr Gabriel Baudouin (an 18th-century Vincentian priest who worked in the slums of Warsaw). In her article about Fr Baudouin she notes with approval, the priest's efforts to encourage the King to grant equal rights to the pupils of the foundling hospital, as to children born within marriage, adding, 'how modern and forward looking was that indefatigable man'. This small outburst of admiration illustrates her deep sense of justice and gives us a brief glimpse into her nursing and socially-based spirituality. It also reminds us of Hanna's spontaneous reaction of suprise and dismay at the way Afro-American patients were being treated in New York City hospitals in the late 1940's, graphically described by Hanna in her memoirs.

It is characteristic of Hanna that nowhere in her papers or correspondence does she refer to a 'road to Damascus experience' or to great 'moments of revelation'. Throughout her life she was extremely quiet about her personal feelings and even quieter about her innermost spiritual thoughts. But there is good reason to believe that the change in Hanna's approach to spirituality and religion was a gradual process over a number of years, a maturation that reflected much thought and quiet introspection. This culminated in her experiences of grief and loss during, and immediately after the Second World War. For Hanna, moral growth and spiritual maturation was not, therefore, an overnight phenomenon: it was a slow development.

In the archives of the Catholic Nurses' Association in Kraków, there is a small missal which was given to Hanna on 24 January 1933 by Mr Wojciech Kluger, with a dedication — *To dear Miss Hanna with a request for prayer.* This would suggest that already by the early 1930's Hanna was happy to receive such a missal and was prepared to pray for its donor. We also know that she used the missal throughout the rest of her life.

Certainly her novels which, as noted, have a semi-autobiographical quality to them, imply that Hanna embarked upon a long road of quiet reflection, rather than a shorter, but more dramatic route of sudden spiritual enlightenment. In her novels Hanna — the narrator — refers to searching for Truth and gradually discovering the meaning and purpose of life. Writing in her autobiographical novel *Blazing Snow,* towards the end of the 1930's she puts into the mouth of one character these words as he looks at a rosary which his friend holds up to him, ' I have no idea how to use it. But if you, my friend… if you trust this, if this is a sign and symbol which you believe in … Since I in turn believe in your honesty, in your inability to lie, I too would like to have one.' In such statements we glimpse the changing attitudes that Hanna was experiencing in her own spiritual life.

But Hanna — the nurse and social activist — spoke very little about how it was that from a position of relative religious indifference and only nominal allegiance to the Catholic Church she came joyfully to affirm her commitment to Catholicism and a Christian gospel-based way of life. Her faith obviously deepened to such an extent that today the Church has acknowledged the heroism of her Christian virtues, and is waiting to formally declare her a saint; an example for all of a holy nurse.

In 1938, Hanna went to Italy with her father, a trip which made an enormous impression on her. Of all the places in Italy that Hanna visited, her stay in Assisi made the greatest impression on her. She would often return to Assisi in her thoughts and reflect upon the beauty of the Umbrian hills. Hanna was overcome by the charm and warmth of Assisi and its charismatic, intense, troubadour saint. The trip confirmed in Hanna her resolve to take matters of spirituality and religion seriously, and she came back from Italy not only energised culturally, but also spiritually uplifted.

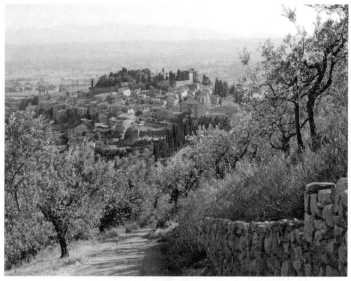

Collection of the author

Assisi

By the outbreak of war in 1939 and most definitely by its con-clusion, Hanna was already a deeply spiritual and reflective woman. Maria Strzembosz, a much younger friend and nursing colleague, who spent some time with Hanna in the USA, commented that there was a quality about Hanna's spirituality at that time, in the late 1940's, which could be interpreted as almost evangelical zeal. She noted that

Hanna had 'a quality about her as if she had just converted from Protestantism to Catholicism'. A similar observation was made by Anna Jabłkowska, a colleague from the WSN. This is interesting because neither before that time nor afterwards would anyone describe Hanna in quite that way. Some of her old friends and colleagues from the WSN actually thought that she had *converted* to Catholicism around this time, so noticeable was her 'religiosity' compared with how they knew her before. What this does confirm about Hanna is that prior to this time she was not known to involve herself *publicly* with religious matters, but that just before, during, and immediately after the war, her pre-occupation and interest in spiritual matters became evident and noticeable.

CHAPTER 7

The Welfare Committee:
Ameliorating the Horrors of War

Where there is hatred let me sow love.
— Attributed to St Francis of Assisi

War broke out in the early hours of 1 September 1939. German troops marched across the Polish plains from the west, and the Luftwaffe dropped bombs on unsuspecting towns and villages. The outbreak of hostilities found Hanna relaxing with her cousin George Zawadzki-Ryźki on his estate near Warsaw. For the second time in her life, a German Front Line prevented Hanna from returning to Kraków and her family.

Hanna was still on her cousin's estate when, on 30 September, she single-handedly rescued an acquaintance — Zofia Nałkowska, a well-known Polish author — from German soldiers who had already set fire to her friend's house. Hanna transported the woman over fifty kilometres in a horse-drawn cart to Dłuźniewa, where Zofia had relatives and was assured of comparative safety. Although Dłuźniewa was not far from Warsaw, it lay across enemy lines and, in the chaotic climate of those first weeks of the war, was a very dangerous undertaking. There was danger not only from divisions of German soldiers, but also from encounters with roaming bands of opportunists, who always seem to accompany the breakdown of social order. This quiet but heroic generosity of spirit was to become typical of Hanna. We only know of this unusual wartime episode because Zofia wrote about it in her autobiography.

Early in the conflict, Hanna experienced several tragedies that no doubt helped her to empathise more intensely with other victims of the war, including many refugees and displaced people whom she was to encounter over the next few years. In September 1939, her cousin Andrew Chrzanowski — with whom she had close ties — was killed during the heroic four-week defence of Warsaw. Her favourite aunt Zofia Szlenkier, who had worked all her life to establish better hospitals and healthcare facilities in Poland, also died in the early days of the war, due in part — ironically — to the appalling conditions in the Warsaw hospitals and inadequate emergency medical coverage. But possibly the most devastating news for Hanna was the death of her close friend from school days, Zofia Wajda, who had worked with her in the Kraków Military Hospital at the end of the First World War and who went on to study medicine while Hanna was studying Polish literature. She died during an enemy attack on the civilian population of Zamość.

By the end of September 1939, the German army had overrun Poland, and Warsaw officially ceased to exist as the capital of independent Poland. The country was forcibly annexed to the Third Reich. The German authorities closed all Polish institutions of learning, including nursing schools, except for the WSN, which managed to function sporadically throughout the war but only as a Red Cross Training Centre. By the middle of October 1939, Hanna had closed her Warsaw apartment and returned to her family in Kraków.

During the autumn of 1939, the Polish army, while fighting the advancing Germans in the west, suddenly faced an unexpected Soviet attack from the east. Thousands of Polish soldiers were taken prisoner by the Russians and sent to Soviet prisoner-of-war camps. Additionally, some soldiers, together with over a million civilians living along the Eastern borders of Poland, were sent to labour camps in Siberia or to other settlements deep inside Soviet territory, such as Kazakhstan and Uzbekistan. Most of the *professional* military officers and government officials who had been sent to POW camps never returned. Hanna's brother Bohdan, an officer in the Reserves, was sent to the Kozielsk POW camp. The vast majority of Polish soldiers who were taken prisoner and sent to Kozielsk camp in 1939, including Hanna's brother, were executed by the Soviets on the express orders of Joseph Stalin. This massacre of soldiers happened in the spring of 1940, in a birch forest near the hamlet of Katyń, not far from Smoleńsk.

By the summer of 1941, when General Anders was allowed to re-form a Polish army in order to help fight the German forces, it became obvious that a large number of Polish officers were unaccounted for. While families at home still lived in hope that their menfolk would eventually return from the camps at the end of the war, Hanna, with her mother and sister-in-law, were never officially told by the Polish Communist authorities what had happened to Bogdan and his fellow officers, despite their repeated requests for information. Bohdan Chrzanowski's body was eventually identified, among the remains of over 10,000 officers found in the mass graves of Katyń. The nature of the atrocity was confirmed through meticulous research conducted by the Germans and the Red Cross, during the war. Doubtless, this was meant to be a political anti-Soviet gesture on the part of the Germans, but at least the facts of the case were revealed and documented fairly soon after the actual event. As well as being a Reserve Officer in the Polish Army, Hanna's brother was a school teacher, a strong family figure, a good brother to Hanna, and a faithful husband.

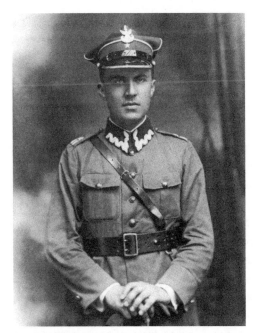

Bohdan Chrzanowski, Hanna's brother who was executed
in the Katyń forests, 1940.

But at the time, in 1940, Hanna and her mother did not know about the atrocity. It took time for the news to emerge, and perhaps, given all the problems they had to overcome just to survive, it was a blessing that, at least for a while, they could hope that Bohdan would eventually return to them. The only communication that they had from Bohdan after he was captured in 1939 came in the form of a card, sent from the Kozielsk POW camp. The card arrived on Christmas Eve 1939. Like many other Polish women in similar circumstances, it was not until much later that they were told informally, in a whisper, of the terrible secret.

Not surprisingly, Hanna and her family were deeply affected. One can well imagine, in these circumstances, why it was subsequently so hard for these women to work *with* the Soviet-backed Communist government, albeit a nominally Polish one. Keeping one's distance from the Polish Communist government seemed to be a natural and appropriate response. Simply knowing that something so awful had happened to so many Polish soldiers, so blatantly contravening the Geneva Convention (which the Soviets never signed anyway), and not to be able to talk publicly about it, must have taken its psychological toll.

Needless to say, because the men were considered to have 'simply disappeared', their wives were never officially treated as war widows and never received compensation from the Soviet Union. To live with this type of knowledge and to be aware of the political lies, without becoming embittered or despairing, takes moral courage and force of character. For Hanna and her mother, however, another more immediate tragedy awaited them.

On 6 November 1939, as part of the German offensive against intellectuals and university professors, code-named *Sonderaktion Krakau*, all the professors at the Jagiellonian University were arrested and deported to Germany. Hanna's father was among the professors who had gathered in the Academic Grand Hall that morning and were sent to Sachsenhausen concentration camp. It was his intense identification with the university which prompted him to show up with his colleagues, even though he had already formally retired from active teaching and in fact, as it later transpired, did not have to be there at all. Writing in a cathartic journal after the death of her husband, Hanna's mother eloquently recounted the harrowing tale of the deception perpetrated that day on the university teaching staff.

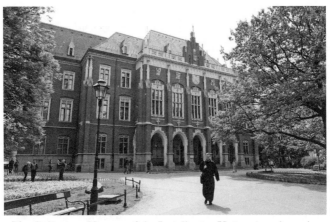

The Collegium Novum of the Jagiellonian University where the professors gathered November 6, 1939.

Hanna's father managed to write a few cards to the family while in captivity, and to the end he was concerned solely about *their* welfare. In turn, he was sent letters and cards by his wife and daughter, albeit censored. Apparently most of their cards were never delivered to him by the camp soldiers. He did not live long in the concentration camp. Brutalised by the conditions in the camp and weakened by the severe regime, he died three months later on 19 January 1940. Hanna and her mother went to Germany to identify his remains and recover the body. They asked for his body to be cremated and then had to wait over a month for the German bureaucracy to forward his ashes to Kraków, for burial. This took place quietly and discreetly on 7 March 1940 in the Rakowicki cemetery, for fear of drawing the attention of the local German authorities to themselves.

The journal written by Hanna's mother tells the disturbing story of their journey to Germany, and it is a strong statement against the brutality of war and its dehumanising effect on young impressionable soldiers. It is written by a sensitive and thoughtful woman, without bitterness, and it is personal and touching, describing how Hanna felt and reacted when they were identifying her father's body. Hanna is portrayed as the supportive daughter, who kept her emotions to herself.

Hanna, in turn, in her own memoir written several decades later, also writes about this trip which took her to wartime Berlin and Oranienburg-Sachsenhausen concentration camp. She vividly recounts the experiences shared with her mother in the concentration camp. Ironically, just three weeks after Dr Chrzanowski's death, those professors who managed to survive the camp ordeal were released, after pressure from Cardinal Sapieha in Kraków and others, and the professors were sent back home. Perhaps, the good professor Chrzanowski was also interceding in heaven on their behalf.

Much has been written about Professor Ignacy Chrzanowski, since he was such a public figure in the university town of Kraków. He knew many people and touched many lives, including as it subsequently turned out, the young student Karol Wojtyła – the future Pope John Paul II. Testaments from professional colleagues and students agree that he had an infectious sense of humour, a remarkable sense of duty and civic responsibility and a passionate loyalty towards his family, his university and his country. His university colleagues recounted how in the concentration camp, when his turn came to deliver a lecture, in spite of his age and weakened condition, he delivered it word-perfect; as his colleagues commented later to his widow, 'and no one went to sleep.' The professors occupied themselves this way in order to stave off boredom and keep their spirits up — an activity more common in POW camps than in concentration camps. Not only did Hanna's father volunteer to give that lecture; he volunteered to deliver a further five, which was more than anyone else in the camp.

Within hours of the arrest of the professors, Hanna and her mother, together with all the other families of academics, were thrown out of their university accommodation to provide living quarters for German officers who had made Kraków their eastern headquarters of the Third Reich. The town was teeming with German soldiers, officials and Nazis; it was probably one of the most dangerous places to be in Poland for dedicated Polish patriots. Hanna and her mother found refuge in an apartment with friends living on Radziwiłłowska Street, where they stayed for the duration of the war.

Thus, in a short space of time, Hanna not only lost members of her close family and her home but was living in an occupied city. Through it all she neither lost her self-control nor displayed anger.

In fact, there is evidence from her close friends that it was precisely during the war that she turned more intensely towards the Church in search of a deeper faith and began to demonstrate a personal witness to the ideals of Christianity, which she now claimed wholeheartedly for herself. For a woman who so unashamedly enjoyed family life and friendship, personal war losses must have been hard to bear. Her deepening spirituality was in no small measure a response to the events which engulfed her; but as we have said, it was also due to her ongoing and deepening friendship and quiet admiration for her deeply religious and socially active friend, Maria Starowieyska. She had known Maria for many years, initially as her nurse-teacher colleague in Kraków, then as a colleague on the nursing journal and now, during the war, as a trusted co-conspirator.

When, in the autumn of 1939, Hanna arrived in Kraków, it was impossible for her to continue her educational work; the occupying forces had also suspended publication of the nursing journal for the duration of the war. Hanna therefore threw herself into social action. Mobilising her community contacts and resources, she turned to taking care of the refugees who were flooding into Kraków. Since there was little war damage in Kraków, the city became a magnet for displaced persons from Warsaw and other devastated towns. Moreover, many refugees were arriving from Poland's eastern border, which was now occupied by the Red Army. People evicted from their homes, were scattered throughout southern Poland; boarding the Lwów to Kraków train, which skirted the entire length of the southern boundary of old Galicia, these internal refugees searched for any safe place along the way to disembark. Additionally, Kraków was becoming filled with Poles whose homes in the north and west of the country had been forcefully taken over by the Nazis in order to rehouse masses of homeless and forcefully uprooted Germans. Thus Kraków was overrun with terrified, lost and bewildered people, often hundreds of miles from their place of birth and homes.

Hanna registered to work with the Polish Welfare Committee (*Polski Komitet Opiekuńczy*), which had been initially set up by Cardinal Sapieha during the First World War. In 1940, the committee was integrated into the Main Benevolent Committee (*Rada Główna Opiekuncza - RGO*). For the rest of the war Hanna worked for the

RGO as the liaison officer between the Kraków branch of the RGO and the German authorities. Her command of the German language not only qualified her for the task, but also helped her to resolve awkward situations with the occupying authorities. Hanna worked for the director of the Kraków RGO – her friend Maria Starowieyska, and later she herself became the director of its home help section, dealing with refugees, displaced persons and orphans. Eventually, she took over the coordination of all social and nursing help for the poor, displaced, or homeless in the Kraków region. The refugees were given material help and accommodation, while an employment exchange was set up and medical care was coordinated, as required.

The scale of the undertaking was phenomenal, and it all took place beneath the eyes of German officials, which made the project even more incredible. Hanna organised a group of volunteers whom she would train and then work with. At the first stage of the project, over three hundred volunteers worked with her. Among the volunteers were registered nurses and unqualified but enthusiastic care workers. For the latter, she organised training sessions and short courses in nursing. Her community nursing friend Aleksandra Dąmbska, living throughout most of the war in Lwów, fulfilled a role similar to Hanna's within the RGO, but in Lwów. The two would communicate with each other whenever there was need for discreet and upon occasion, clandestine help. These pioneer nurses together with Maria Starowieyska were now prepared, at great personal cost, to completely commit themselves to social action and emergency relief work. They fully justified the trust that was placed in them.

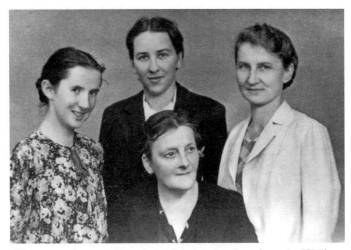

Hanna standing on the right with her co-workers from the Welfare Committee (RGO) with Maria Starowiejska in the centre bottom.

With Maria Starowieyska, Hanna worked to satisfy the material needs of the refugees, while also taking care of their psychological and spiritual wellbeing. Hanna was particularly concerned for the welfare of women and children. She coordinated foster care for children who became separated from their parents and for war orphans. Among these many thousands of children were those of Jewish descent. These too she would place with substitute families and with various orders of nuns who ran orphanages in the Kraków area. In the Kraków region alone, at least thirteen religious houses are known to have sheltered Jewish children. Such clandestine activity was forbidden by the German authorities. If they had discovered that she was shielding and protecting Jewish children, she ran the risk not only of being executed herself; indeed, her entire workforce faced the same risk. It is probably one of the most difficult ethical decisions ever to make — whether to risk saving the life of one child at the possible expense of many other lives.

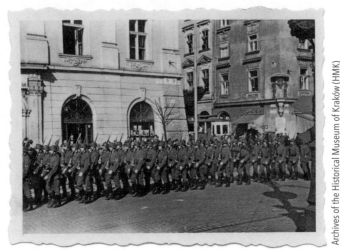

German soldiers in Kraków old town square

Little is known about the clandestine activities of Hanna Chrzanowska during the war. We know that she was involved in various
secret and illegal activities, but to this day only a few of her wartime
actions have been reliably documented. Janina Porębska, who had
given shelter in her apartment on Radziłłowska Street to Hanna and
her mother for the duration of the war, recounts how one afternoon,
Hanna arrived somewhat earlier than usual from work at the Welfare committee, and when asked why she was so white and shaking
and not her usual cheerful self, Hanna answered in one of those rare
moments of being caught off guard, that she had just come back from
accompanying a little Jewish girl across the whole of Kraków, to a
safe house, and added, 'and you could tell from a mile away that she
was Jewish'. But such slips were rare. In fact, few people knew about
Hanna's work protecting and sheltering Jews. Hanna left no record of
what was going through her mind or how she felt as she made those
dangerous decisions, and except for some hastily-written biographical
notes about the children who were being placed in foster homes, in
order to make it easier for others to later reconnect these children with
their families after the war, there is no written evidence of what took
place. For everyone's safety and protection it was important to leave as
little evidence as possible.

Apart from Maria Starowieyska, another nurse who is known to have made similar decisions was her old friend and co-worker in Lwów, Aleksandra Dąmbska, who in 2010 was posthumously awarded the title *Righteous Among the Nations*, by the Israeli government, and whose name is now inscribed in the Yad Vashem memorial. Aleksandra remarked to her family after the war that she considered her actions to be a natural consequence of all that she believed in; that is, in order to be true to herself, she could not have done otherwise than to rescue others. Hanna subscribed to the same beliefs. The children whom Hanna sought to protect did not know who had placed them with their new families or in safe orphanages. Neither did the institutions and families ask probing questions. It was vital for the success of Hanna's clandestine work that she be considered by the Germans to be above reproach.

With Maria Starowieyska, Hanna also organised summer 'camps' for youngsters in the houses and mansions of the landed gentry around the Kraków region. Róża Kieniewicz, who worked for a while with the RGO committee in Kraków, stated in the 1990's, from her post-war home in Perth, Scotland, that she remembered well those summer 'outings' and camps held at her parental home (a sizeable manor house) in Wójczy, which were organised for orphaned and destitute children. Other pre-war Małopolska landowners have since come forward and recounted their stories for the postulator of Hanna's canonisation case, about these children's camps, including some of the children who were cared for (now elderly individuals), and whom she was trying to 'feed up'. Some children needed extra nutrition as they were severely malnourished. Somehow, even in war-torn and impoverished Kraków, Hanna managed to set up a Nutrition Bank with the support of her friends and contacts among the landed gentry. Food and milk from the farms was provided for the sick and those who were in greatest need. For a few months in 1942 Hanna even undertook to work extra shifts on the neonatal unit of the medical centre in Kraków, working alongside a German doctor in order to ensure that the care he delivered was safe and that he, as a consultant on the ward, was not practising euthanasia on Polish infants.

As the war dragged on, she added to her ever-increasing work load the visiting of prisoners in the Montelupich Prison. Her friend

Aleksandra Dąmbska worked in a similar capacity in Lwów. Their knowledge of German and their neutral status as healthcare workers put them in an excellent position to note who the prisoners were and how long they had been there. Much of this important information was subsequently conveyed to the Resistance in the underground Home Army. According to Aleksandra, this 'extension' of their welfare committee work evolved naturally, since it was also part of their remit to deliver Red Cross parcels to the prisoners and to convey prisoners' letters to relatives and friends. Alexandra recounted years later that she would carry back encrypted messages with information for the Polish Resistance in the contaminated laundry of prisoners with tuberculosis.

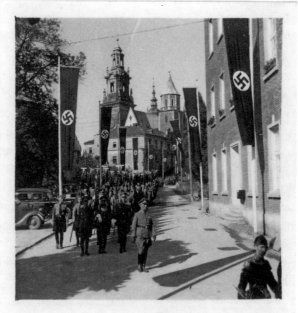

German soldiers marching down from Wawel Castle Wawel Castle. General Franck made his headquarters in Kraków for the duration of the war.

Hanna was so good at covering her tracks that today we still do not know whether she was officially part of the clandestine, underground Home Army resistance movement or not, and what was the exact nature of her relationship with them. We do know however, that Maria Starowieyska was an active and trusted member of the resistance and was arrested more than once by the gestapo. The last time was in November 1944, when the German soldiers arrested her directly from the offices of the RGO, in front of terrified volunteers. After brutal interrogation, they sent her to Ravensbrük concentration camp. She miraculously survived the camp, and died shortly after the war in Kraków in 1951, in an orphanage for destitute children and single mothers, which she had helped to establish before the war. One of her brothers died in Dachau concentration camp in 1941 and was beatified in 1999 by Pope St John Paul II, as a martyr, together with other Polish victims of Nazism. Maria came from a family with a strong Christian tradition and so it is not surprising that she had such a profound influence on Hanna's growth in faith.

Throughout the war, Hanna organised the delivery of medicines and nursing supplies to the wounded soldiers of the Home Army. She also hid allied soldiers and Polish Resistance fighters in hospitals, clinics and monasteries around the town. For example, she was involved in hiding some English soldiers on the run from the Germans, placing them on the infectious disease ward of Professor Józef Kostrzewski. Allied soldiers were also hidden among the homeless and destitute seeking refuge in the Capuchin Monastery on Loretańska Street, which functioned at the time like many other convents, as a centre for those who were homeless and displaced on account of the war.

During the Warsaw uprising towards the end of the war (1 August to 3 October 1944), Hanna delivered medicines to beleaguered hospitals and first-aiders, travelling to Warsaw several times by train. After the heroic but abortive uprising, a new wave of refugees arrived in Kraków, and again Hanna was in the difficult position of trying to accommodate them and provide for their basic needs. Not only did she look after the refugees who managed to escape from the burning city of Warsaw, but she sent a few nurses who travelled several times to the transit refugee camp of Pruszków, outside Warsaw, to help the homeless people of Warsaw. Having marched the civilian population out of the ruined city, the Germans placed them all in this camp. The refugees were in despair, their spirits broken. They were homeless, as the capital of Poland now lay in ruins.

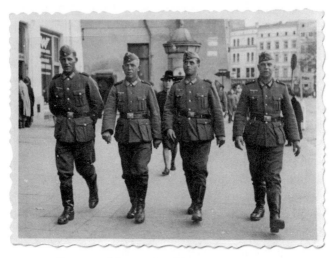

German soldiers in the old town square, 1941.

CHAPTER 8

A Profession Enslaved: The Post-War Years

*'Without freedom of thought,
there can be no such thing as wisdom...'*
— Benjamin Franklin

With the conclusion of the war in 1945, Hanna undertook to work with the United Nations Refugee Relief Agency (UNRRA) in Kraków, continuing to organise and distribute aid to refugees. At the same time, the town authorities assigned her and her mother a flat on Łobzowska Street. Located opposite a monastery of Carmelite nuns, this replaced the large pre-war apartment that had been requisitioned by the Germans, but it enabled them to move out of their temporary (wartime) quarters on Radziwiłłowska Street. Sometime after the death of her mother in 1951, moved by the desperate plight of a homeless family, Hanna gave them the use of the flat, reserving one small room for herself. Many such quiet gestures of solidarity with the poor and homeless were unknown to her contemporaries and nursing colleagues; they came to light only after Hanna's death.

After the war, the schools of nursing reopened, and Hanna naturally went back to work at the Kraków School of Nursing, where the first post-war Principal was Miss Anna Rydlówna (1884-1969). Fortunately, Miss Rydlówna knew Hanna well, and had worked with her before the war. She admired her community nursing work and fully supported Hanna's programmes and projects. Anna Rydlówna had been active in Kraków educating nurses together with Maria Epstein (as we have seen, later Servant of God Sister Magdalena OP — now a candidate for sainthood), and like Hanna had been sent to many countries in Europe and to North America to examine the education and working practices of nurses — mostly through the beneficence of the Rockefeller Foundation. Hanna occupied the position of

vice-principal and was given responsibility for coordinating community nursing placements and lecturing on community nursing. She
personally set up and directed the department, which specialised in
home care for the chronically ill.

During the immediate post-war years the School of Nursing
functioned much as it had prior to the war, except that the programme
of study, which before the war had been two years, was lengthened to
three. This unusual move (unique to Kraków) was due to concern over
the lower quality of wartime education of the young women — as
secondary schools had been closed by the Germans for the duration of
the war — and not because of any desire to upgrade nurses' education.
The first post-war entrants into nursing tended to be mature women
who had wished to become nurses but whose educations had been
interrupted by the war. Many had already attended short emergency
nurse training courses and had completed various Red Cross courses,
while quite a few had worked as volunteers in field hospitals and relief
centres. All of them had witnessed more during the war years than
was strictly necessary for their maturation and healthy development.
These enthusiastic women had been hardened by the war; indeed they
must have been extremely practical just to survive it. Hanna wrote in
her memoirs that it had been a pleasure to work with these women,
despite the material difficulties that they all faced at that time. Hanna
introduced these students to community nursing, focusing on visits to
the chronically ill, some of whom had had neither visitors nor medical
help for years.

Unexpectedly, in 1946, Hanna had the good fortune to be one
of several Polish nurses who were awarded a UNRRA scholarship
to travel to the USA to study the development of community/home
nursing; in fact she was the group co-ordinator. She therefore missed
some of the uglier aspects of the reorganisation of the Kraków School
of Nursing and was out of the country during a period which was
politically very difficult for Poland. The scholarship came at just the
right moment.

The study trip was seriously delayed due to red tape — the large
amount of paperwork which needed to be processed before the group
could finally obtain the necessary visas and documents. In this uncer-
tain climate, Hanna left earlier than the rest of the group and went

on to London with a small group of nurses waiting for the rest to join them. Meanwhile, Hanna polished her rather rusty English, visited museums, attended concerts and bemoaned the quality of the cakes in Lyons tea shops. Eventually the other nurses left for Paris, where they spent another six weeks studying English in the mornings, and sightseeing the city in the afternoons, while waiting for their necessary papers and for transport to the USA. For a time, the nurses expected to sail any day from Le Havre, but the French merchant navy was on strike, and so in the end they had to travel to the USA via England and not by ship as originally planned, but by plane.

The nurses stayed in the USA for almost a year. As was always the case in such circumstances, one of them was a political spy. It is a testament to Hanna's equanimity that this woman was never isolated or made to feel left out. Neither could the woman ever find anything negative to say about the nurses! They went to the USA to observe modern methods of nursing, and that was exactly what they did.

Initially, they were based on Staten Island, New York, where there was at that time a large United States Public Health Service Hospital [USPHSH], the largest in the USA, where patients with various infectious and tropical diseases were looked after. There was also an impressive health and community education outreach programme attached to the hospital. Moreover, a large asylum, the Willowbrook State School, had been built just before the war and while during the war and in the late 1940s it had been taken over for the care of American veterans and soldiers, shortly afterwards it became an asylum for children and adults with learning difficulties and severe handicaps. While the Polish nurses were on Staten Island, it still would have functioned as a form of Veterans' Hospital. Later however, it became infamous as a place where unorthodox medical practices were conducted and for the appalling care of its vulnerable residents. When the Polish nurses were placed on Staten Island in late 1946, they probably were based at and worked from the USPHSH, but they also visited other hospitals and medical establishments around the island.

While on Staten Island, some of the nurses became disgruntled, feeling that too much work was being imposed on them. Maria Strzembosz recalls Hanna remonstrating with them, stating: 'If you had been given the chance to visit America at the price of peeling potatoes, would you not have leapt at the opportunity? Well, is it not the same with us? If nothing else enjoy your trip and try to learn even from the small insignificant things that you are observing'. Members of the group remembered what she said, even after many years. Hanna encouraged the nurses to visit the sights of New York, go to theatres, attend concerts and visit museums. She certainly enjoyed the cultural side of the visit herself. One can hear in her advice offered to the younger nurses, echoes of the encouragement given to the exuberant young Hanna in Paris — prompting the nurses to avail themselves of all the opportunities that the trip presented to them.

During their stay in the USA they also made contact with the local Polish-American community, and Hanna was asked to deliver a speech in New Jersey to the Polish Americans.

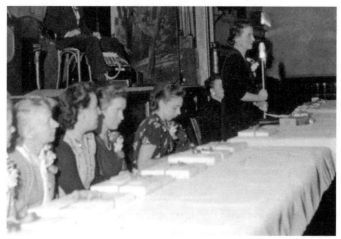

Hanna (standing) giving a talk in New Jersey to Polish Americans.

Once, they were invited to talk to a local American church group about their experiences in war-torn Europe, but the cultural and educational gulf between the women was so great that the American women laughed at them and were amused at some of the stories. The Polish nurses decided not to accept such invitations again. Hanna, the quintessential diplomat and the quiet spokesperson for the group, agreed that it was too embarrassing for the Polish nurses to consider repeating the event.

At some point during their stay, the group moved up Manhattan Island to Washington Heights, where they were based at Maxwell Hall. This was the Nurses' home and base for the School of Nursing attached to Columbia Presbyterian Hospital, now part of Columbia University and renamed Columbia Presbyterian University Medical Centre. It was an imposing Edwardian building, poised on the high escarpment of the Hudson River, offering a panoramic view of New Jersey and the George Washington Bridge. The view was to impress many generations of nurses, not only the Polish visitors. This purpose-built institution, modelled on the best nursing schools in London, was to fascinate Hanna. Sadly for social historians and historians of healthcare architecture, but of great benefit to current patients and nursing students, it has been pulled down and replaced by a modern state-of-the-art medical and nursing campus.

Hanna and her colleagues were enchanted by the physical location and architecture of the nursing school. They were even more impressed by the authority and dignity of the Director of Maxwell Hall, Miss Florence Vanderbilt, who would stand at the hospital entrance every morning to check that the nurses were ready and prepared for the day's work. In Poland, the positions of Director of the Nurses' Home and of hospital Matron were not so well developed, and it must have amused and impressed the Polish nurses to observe the activities of the hospital matron and subsequent director of the nursing school, Miss Elizabeth Gill.

Hanna's study visits took her to Harlem, where she worked and observed nursing care being delivered to the poor and indigent, and particularly to members of the black community. The blatant racism of America in the late 1940's was evident even in the healthcare field, and made a strong impression on the Polish women. The obvious separation of blacks and whites shocked the Polish nurses; they commented upon it amongst themselves and noted it in their diaries. Hanna wrote years later about accompanying on her rounds a black district nurse who was doing home visits. She recalled her as being 'wonderful and wise', while others of the group remembered the effect on the black patients of the nursing administrations of Hanna and the other Polish nurses. Some of these patients said that they had never before been touched by a white woman and were greatly moved by the care these

Polish nurses gave them. Hanna vowed then and there, based on what she saw in the USA, to work towards setting up district (visiting) nursing in Poland.

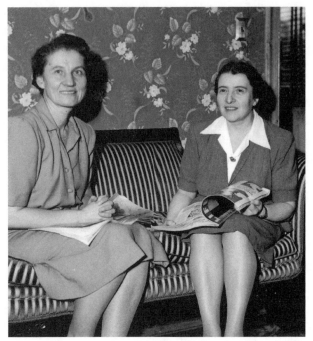

Hanna (on the left) with Maria Pągowska in New York City, 1946.

When the time came for the study programme to end, alone of the whole group of UNRRA nurses (there were also Czechoslovak, Chinese and Italian nurses in the programme), the Polish group was eager to get back home. Excited by what they had seen and experienced, they could not wait to get back to work in Poland, even though they were aware of the difficult political times ahead in their home country and the vastness of the task that awaited them. The non-Polish nurses cried and pleaded to remain in America, but the Poles had work to do and wanted to start as soon as possible. The group returned to Europe on the Danish ship Jutlandia, which after a few years was requisitioned by the Red Cross for use as a hospital ship during the Korean War.

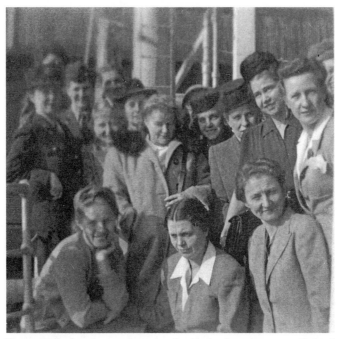

Hanna (right hand corner) on the ship Jutlandia returning to Poland.

One cannot but wonder to what extent the patriotic and pragmatic influence of Hanna was at work during the nurses' stay in New York. The visit to America must have been such an enormous culture shock for them after the deprivations of war. Hanna comments that the stay in New York City confirmed her in her conviction that 'community nursing demands wise practice, takes in many aspects of life and, as with other nursing disciplines, demands a high level of preparation and training'.

CHAPTER 9

Being an Apostle:
Life in the Polish People's Republic

If we, with the help of God, do our duty and work for His honour
and glory, no one will interfere with us.
— St Marianna Cope

Back in Poland, Hanna returned to her work at the Kraków School of Nursing. In the new political climate, it was inevitable that the School, which had always been patriotic and strongly religious, would be forced to change its orientation. Its distinguished principal, Miss Anna Rydlówna, was a devout practising Catholic, which was considered politically unacceptable in a Communist country for a person in her position of authority. Furthermore, during the war she had been a member of the Resistance. For these reasons the new authorities perceived Anna Rydlówna as being essentially anti-socialist and working against the Communist government's objectives for the new secular Polish nation.

Immediately after the war, a quiet civil war was waged between the Soviet-imposed Polish Communists and members of the old pre-war order. The latter included Resistance groups of the former Home Army, that is, soldiers who had not surrendered their weapons at the end of the war. The continued presence of Polish resistance fighters was a sore point with Polish Communists, who identified resistance members (mostly wartime underground Home Army soldiers) with supporters of Marshall Józef Piłsudzki and members of the Free Polish Army led by Generals Anders and Maczek. Both of these generals had been based outside Poland for most of the war and their soldiers, after fighting with the allies, had been demobilised in Great Britain and in the main refused to return to a Communist Poland.

In this manner between 1946 and 1954, Poland was in the grip of a power struggle, whose greatest casualties were the returning soldiers of the Polish Army, Roman Catholic clergy, demobilised resistance fighters, landed gentry and aristocracy, pre-war academics and members of the *intelligentsia*. Anyone who opposed, or who was thought to oppose, Socialist Communist ideology was persecuted. Such individuals were systematically imprisoned and tortured; a few were subsequently released, physically broken and their health permanently ruined. Many more died in captivity and were never heard of again. Only after the fall of Communism in 1989 would historians and social commentators begin to write and talk about that tragic period and begin to collate the horrifying evidence against the Socialist ruling party.

Even directors of schools of nursing were not exempt from political harassment and scrutiny by the secret police – the so called *Urząd Bezpieczeństwa* or UB. The secret police's frequent visits to the nursing school in Kraków began to negatively influence the atmosphere in that institution. Nursing students were interrogated, threatened and even kept in prison cells, albeit for short periods of time. In 1949, Miss Rydlówna was forced to retire from her position as director of the school along with her vice-principal, Teresa Kulczyńska, a close friend, co-editor and great supporter of Hanna's work. Teresa (1894-1992) was one of the first registered nurses to work in Poland, after gaining her nursing qualifications in Boston, Massachusetts and at Columbia University in New York City prior to the opening of the Warsaw School of Nursing. She was also one of the first Polish recipients of a Rockefeller scholarship. At this time the School was separated from the Jagiellonian University, nationalised and, upon becoming a state-run nursing school, taken over by the Ministry of Health.

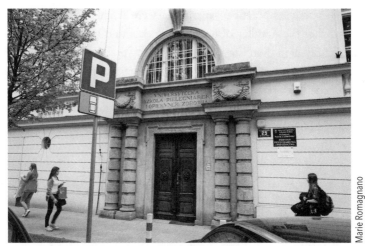

Krakow University School of Nursing

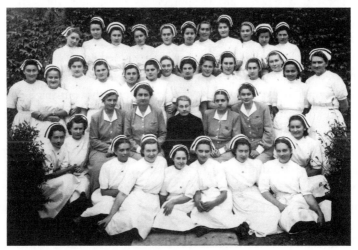

Hanna sitting to the left of the Director of the school of nursing,
Anna Rydlówna (in black).

Although all nursing lecturers had to attend Socialist indoctrina-
tion sessions delivered by special 'education officers' of the Communist
Party, no one stopped Hanna from conducting her own community
exercises or delivering her own courses to the students. However, the
duration of the new nursing programme was reduced to two years
after the short trial period of having it last three years. This meant

that the students' practical experiences were seriously curtailed. It also meant that the number of nursing students that could look after the chronically ill in their homes on community practice was substantially reduced, which in turn affected the home help nursing structure that Hanna had so laboriously set up. On top of these adverse changes, the new principal of the school, Miss Zofia Kurkowa, was not particularly fond of Hanna, nor sympathetic to the need for community nursing.

By all accounts Zofia Kurkowa was an amazing woman. Those who worked with her, or who attended the School during her director-ship, reported that she could be something of an embarrassment to the School's reputation, although the education authorities at the Ministry of Health considered her to be an efficient nurse administrator, and she did have the necessary managerial and nursing qualifications to lead the school of nursing. She had an exemplary war record and had proved to be personally accountable and courageous. Interestingly, at the conclusion of the war, upon the liberation of Auschwitz concentration camp at the end of January 1945, she volunteered to set up nursing care in the camp's main newly established hospital for the sick and traumatised survivors. But, unfortunately, she also developed serious personality problems (today we would probably put them down to post-traumatic stress disorder), which were to become increasingly evident, not only to staff and work colleagues, but even the students.

Some students recall how she would routinely greet the students in the morning from the top of the stairs, in hair-curlers and a dressing gown with her favourite pet dog under her arm — a far cry from the prim professionalism of the principal at Columbia Presbyterian School of Nursing in New York City, who was so admired by Hanna. The students and staff were also disturbed by some of Miss Kurkowa's more questionable habits, such as feeding her dog off plates from the students' dining-room, an unhygienic practice which called into question her level of understanding in regards to matters of public health. Although possibly a minor point, this was something that upset the students considerably — and one they still remember.

Miss Kurkowa also swore profusely at students and staff when she was annoyed — which was apparently quite often. The difference between this principal and the gentle and genteel Anna Rydlówna, could not have been greater. It is significant that Hanna was never known to complain about the principal, and certainly not in front of students or fellow staff members, even when as vice-principal, she had to rectify the mistakes of her superior.

There are several nurses alive today who recall Hanna during this period (1948 to 1955), when she was a nursing instructor and vice-principal at the school of nursing. Some of those nursing students became Hanna's close friends and co-workers, including Helena Matoga (who was to become the vice-postulator of Hanna's cause for canonisation) and the late Irena Iżycka, while others went on to work with Hanna on the parish nursing project, such as Wacława Bogdal and Alina Rumun. They all recall Hanna as being very knowledgeable, practical and above all a caring individual. They remember to this day her concern for their well-being and their mental and spiritual welfare.

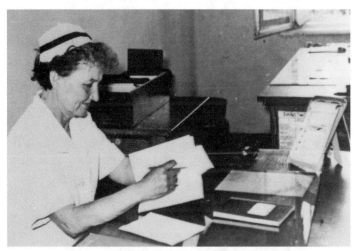

Hanna at work in her office in the School of Nursing.

They recall how one May, during *Juvenalia* (the Jagiellonian University students' ancient rite of passage, celebrated with much partying), the nursing students wanted to stay out after 11pm in order to be present in the town square at midnight, when the result of the contest for the most beautiful woman was to be announced. Ever hopeful of winning, the students wished to enter into the spirit of the activities, but nursing school regulations forbade the students from staying out after 10pm. Despite the prevailing political climate, in which the students and staff could have been dismissed from the school on the most fragile of pretexts, Hanna gave permission to the students to stay out late, provided they all came back by 1am and did nothing that would reflect badly on the school. This incident demonstrates at least two aspects of the relationship between the students and Hanna. Firstly, they trusted her enough to tell her what they were planning to do, and they knew that she would not laugh at them, nor deny their wishes out of hand. Secondly, it shows that Hanna was prepared to bend the rules. Hanna knew that this particular request meant a lot to the young students and that their psychological well-being was more important at that moment than any rules and regulations.

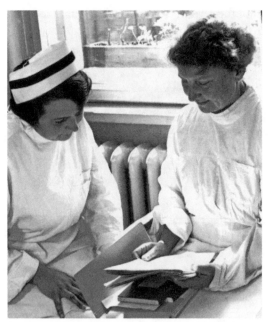

Hanna with a colleague in the Kraków School of Nursing, 1950s

Helena Matoga recalls how one Christmas Eve she and some of her friends were scheduled to work the Christmas shifts in the hospital. The Polish custom of celebrating Christmas Eve with a special evening meal called *Wigilia,* is an old and sacred tradition. The meal has the emotional and religious overtones of the Jewish *Seder,* or Passover meal, and the homeliness and warmth of the American family-centred feast of Thanksgiving, but conducted in the joyful context of Christmas. Even during deprivations of war or in Soviet gulags or German concentration camps, wherever Poles were to be found, the feast of *Wigilia* was always kept or attempts were made to keep it, even by atheists!

Imagine the situation of the young nursing students, away from home for the first time, in a political environment where no religious or even secular feast was acknowledged by the Communists, where Christmas Day was considered to be just another working day, and therefore no decorations, cribs or carols were allowed on the wards, or anywhere else in the hospital – the homesickness, nostalgia and hurt must have been overwhelming.

Helena tells the story of how she walked slowly and reluctantly into the school dining-room, despondent. There, in front of her, was the smiling figure of Hanna dressed for the occasion; the tables were festively set; a crib and a candlelit Christmas tree stood in an alcove. Hanna looked at Helena and her friends, embraced them all warmly and, after allowing them to shed a few tears, proceeded to hurry them up, to change out of their uniforms and start celebrating *Wigilia*, the ancient Polish Christmas Eve feast.

This initiative did not come from the school administration or the Principal — it was something Hanna had organised herself. It is yet more evidence of Hanna's concern for the students' welfare and of her courage. To go ahead with the celebration in the certain knowledge of political repercussions and that she would be accused of 'leading the youth astray with anti-socialist activities' took nerve and determination. It also says something about the powers of persuasion that Hanna must have had among her peers, for even if she instigated the surprise feast, many others must have been involved. To this day, Helena recalls that Christmas Eve with emotion and awareness of the personal cost to Hanna that this escapade must have involved.

In a country where over a third of all healthcare workers had died during the war, Hanna was professionally respected and held in high regard. Communist officials could not afford to ignore her talents and her wealth of knowledge, and so she was allowed to conduct continuing professional education courses for qualified nurses. She ran a methodological course for nursing educators to teach community nursing skills, at the state-run nurse educators training institute,

Państwowa Szkoła Instruktorska, in Warsaw. In 1950 she was asked by the Ministry of Health to conduct a survey into the state of community nursing services and programmes in Poland. Hanna personally conducted the research and drew up a report for the Minister.

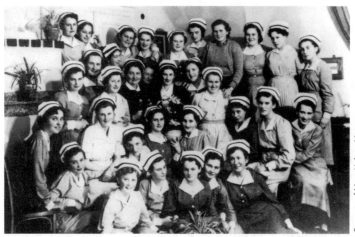

Hanna surrounded by her last intake of students, including H. Matoga – currently Vice-postulator of Hanna's canonisation cause. Kraków, 1956.

But Hanna was a practising Catholic, attending daily Mass and actively participating in the religious life of Kraków diocese. This, however, for the Communist government was bound to be seen as defiant and counter-revolutionary activity. It is no wonder that the authorities wanted her removed from her position of influence among students; they just were not sure how to go about it. In 1957 they demanded that she stop teaching at the Kraków School of Nursing. They asked her instead to become Director of the School of Psychiatric Nursing at the country's largest psychiatric hospital, located in Kobierzyn about seven miles from the centre of Kraków. They did not tell her that no one else wanted the post. One can only presume that the authorities were confident either that Hanna would not take up the post, or that, if she did, her 'negative' influence on nursing students there would be much diminished. The move was intended to humiliate Hanna, but even in Kobierzyn, she managed to leave her mark.

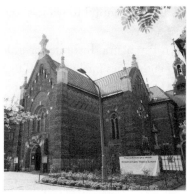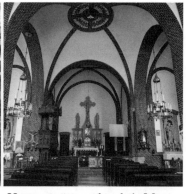

Marie Romagnano

Carmelite Monastery Chapel where Hanna participated in daily Mass. It is situated across the street from Hanna's apartment. Hanna's funeral Mass was celebrated in this chapel.

She did influence the students there, and they fondly remember the time when they worked with her. For the authorities, the final straw came when Hanna allowed some of her psychiatric nursing students to join the second nursing pilgrimage to Jasna Góra in 1957, to pay homage to the icon of the Black Madonna at the National Shrine of Our Lady of Częstochowa. The first national pilgrimage of nurses to Częstochowa took place in 1956, and its main organiser was Teresa Strzembosz, the sister-in-law of Maria Strzembosz, Hanna's younger colleague and friend with whom she had worked while on her UNNRA scholarship in the USA. Teresa was an energetic and committed Catholic social worker from Warsaw. The nurses' pilgrimage was to become an annual event, continuing to this day.

It would appear that Hanna and Teresa met for the first time in Częstochowa during that 1956 pilgrimage. They had much to say to each other concerning community health care and one common interest which they talked about at length was the need to establish some form of community nursing aimed at the chronically sick and housebound frail elderly. In spite of their age difference, their friendship continued and several years later Hanna was to help Teresa set up Parish Nursing in Warsaw. Interestingly, the diocese of Warsaw has recently declared that Teresa Strzebosz can be given the title of Servant of God and the cause for her canonisation has been formally opened. As noted already, this wonderful communion of saints, so evident during the course of Hanna's life, is beautiful to witness, and has brought forth great fruit and much joy.

Hanna worked at the Kobierzyn Psychiatric Institute for little more than a year, because the Socialist authorities finally decided that the best way to deal with her was in fact to close down the School of Nursing. Hanna was dismissed from her post, and in 1958 she took early retirement. For the first time in over thirty years she was no longer working as a salaried professional nurse. Paradoxically, the current Managing Director of Kobierzyn Psychiatric Hospital, Mr Stanisław Kracik, is familiar with Hanna and her work. He first came across Hanna as a young university student, when he was involved with her Parish Nursing movement in Kraków, as one of her many young student volunteers. There is now a plaque in the hospital chapel commemorating Hanna's activities and presence in that institution.

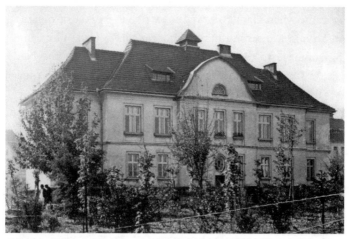

Main building of Kobierzyn Hospital before the Second World War

CHAPTER 10

Deeper Conversion to Christ:
A Benedictine Oblate

'Solitude is the very ground from which community grows.'
— Henri Nouwen

Hanna was already a committed Catholic when she began to visit the Benedictine Abbey of Tyniec, located outside Kraków on a picturesque cliff overlooking a wide bend of the Wisła River (the Vistula). According to Dom Leon Knabit OSB, now an elderly monk at the abbey, who was a friend and confessor to Hanna from her first visits to the monastic community around 1951, Hanna knew the entire Mass by heart, both in Latin and in Polish. She was also well-acquainted with other liturgical texts, with many biblical passages and most gospel readings, from which she would often quote. Before showing serious interest in Benedictine spirituality, Hanna already attended Mass daily, and after the war, when Hanna lived across the road from a monastery of Carmelite nuns, she often joined them for early morning Mass.

Hanna started going to Tyniec at a time when she felt particularly bereft of human support. Both her mother and long-standing friend Maria Starowieyska died in 1951, and the shock of the dark realities of Stalinist-dominated Polish Communism of the 1950s, must have weighed heavily on her heart.

Tyniec Abbey was originally a medieval foundation of 1044 which, like other monastic establishments, had been dissolved by the occupying Austrian authorities in 1816. After much effort and prayer, the ancient foundation was re-established in 1928 with the arrival of Dom Charles van Oost from the Belgian Abbey of St André in Zevenkerken. Prior to his arrival, Belgian Benedictines from the Abbey of St André and from the Benedictine foundations of Bueron

113

in Germany and Solesmes in France also played a role in fostering the spirit of St Benedict in Poland, thus preparing the groundwork for the formal return of the monks to Tyniec. This occurred just a month before the outbreak of the Second World War. Dom Charles was the first Prior of the newly re-established foundation and continued to forge close ties with the "parent" Belgian Abbey of St André. Tyniec Priory did not obtain the title and privileges of an independent abbey until 1969.

Throughout the Second World War, the newly re-established foundation continued to function. It also grew in spiritual importance and scholarly reputation, despite some damage to the buildings and the dispersion of many of the monks — several of whom were martyred in Dachau concentration camp. A number of the Tyniec monks were associated with post-conciliar liturgical reforms in Poland. Some were active members of the Polish Bishops' liturgy commission and helped to produce a new translation of the Bible – the first Polish translation since that produced by Fr Jakub Wujek S.J. in the seventeenth century.

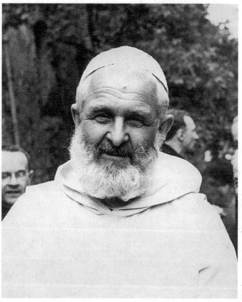

With permission of Tyniec Abbey

Dom Piotr Rostworowski, OSB

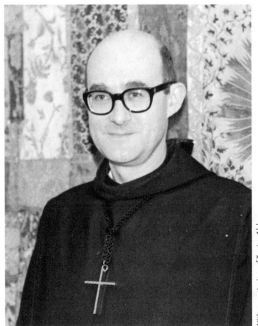

With permission of Tyniec Abbey

Dom Placyd Galiński, OSB

Monks from Tyniec became renowned biblical scholars. Dom
Placid Galiński, who was the first formally elected abbot of the
re-erected Tyniec foundation (and was abbot from 1969 to 1977),
translated the Divine Office into Polish and put Polish words to liturgical chants. He was a good friend of Hanna and at one point became
Hanna's spiritual director. The monks engaged in academic scholarship
in areas of historical research, scripture studies and philosophy and
held various academic posts at the Pontifical Theological Academy in
Kraków. They also taught at the various seminaries in Kraków.

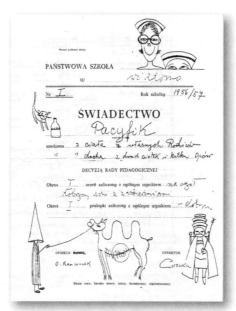

An end of year 'report' prepared for the prior of Tyniec, Dom Placyd
Galiński, by Hanna – as a joke. Dom Placyd was Hanna's spiritual
director for a while. Note Hanna's self-caricature with a tiara of nursing
caps in the lower right-hand corner… It is signed *Cioteczka* – Auntie.

Meanwhile, Dom Piotr Rostworowski (1910-1999), was elected
the second prior at Tyniec Abbey from 1951 to 1959, at the very
time that Hanna started going there, and was one of her first spiritual directors, as well as being spiritual director to Fr Karol Wojtyła.
He was also appointed Visitor to the monks at the nearby Camaldolese Hermitage of Bielany, which is visible from the Tyniec abbey
escarpments. Dom Piotr Rostworowski was a famed spiritual director
and scholar, and in 1968 Bishop Karol Wojtyła and the Benedictine
authorities in Rome asked him to help re-vitalise the local community
of Camaldolese hermits. It speaks volumes for the spiritual stature
and sacrificial nature of Dom Piotr Rostworowski and the powers of
persuasion of Bishop Wojtyła that Dom Peter left the relative security
and friendship of his Tyniec Benedictine community and adopted the
spirituality of a Camaldolese hermit in order to assist the Camaldolese.
He died in Italy, and was revered for his holiness.

Hanna felt sufficiently drawn to this particularly vibrant, prayerful and scholarly Benedictine foundation, that in 1957 she made a

vow to live in association with the Abbey as a Benedictine oblate. The promise Hanna made as an oblate of Tyniec Abbey, before the whole monastic community, in the presence of Dom Piotr the prior, with a signed document as testament to her commitment placed on the high altar, and entrusted to the abbey's care, included a promise to embrace what St Benedict called in his Rule '*conversatio morum*', or conversion of manners.

She chose Clare as her oblate name, after the companion of Francis of Assisi, who established the monastery of St Damian (a redundant Benedictine priory given to St Francis), where she cared for Francis near the end of his life, and where he composed the 'Canticle of the Sun.' Hanna had not forgotten her admiration for the two poor saints of Assisi and their dedication to restoring vitality to the Church through lives of prayer, poverty and simplicity. Towards the end of her life, Hanna was known also to lead a simple, basic lifestyle, while managing always to look elegant.

The writer Esther de Waal, a contemporary Anglican Benedictine oblate, interprets *coversatio* as meaning '...to respond totally and integrally to the word of Christ sent to all of us: "Come, follow me!" ' (*Seeking God: The Way of St Benedict*, p 53.) Hanna took this promise seriously and at face value, truly opening herself to Christ and determined to follow his call; without looking back or counting the cost. One could almost say, that it was her Benedictine promise which started to determine and ultimately shape the Christocentric nature of the next twenty years of her life. These were the years of pastoral activity for which she is best remembered, and most widely known. Hanna's life from this time onwards was considered by many people who knew her to be one of holiness.

In a brochure given to prospective applicants enquiring about becoming an oblate, the oblate master of St John's Abbey, Minnesota wrote that '*oblates shape their lives by living the wisdom of Christ as interpreted by St Benedict...[they] strive to become holy in their chosen way of life.*' That is precisely what Hanna took to heart. She remained a committed community nurse but now with a renewed focus and passion, she also strove to follow Christ, and to seek him out, in the form of the marginalised and abandoned. That is, she strove to be holy, and took as her inspiration and practical guidance in this task the Rule of St

Benedict. Abbott Charles van Oost — who restored the Benedictines to Tyniec — used to say that Benedictine spirituality consisted of one hundred per cent New Testament living: so therefore let us try and simply be Christians [people of the Gospel] in this place to which the Lord has called us. Something of this simple Benedictine call to live the gospel life resonated deep within Hanna's soul.

Hanna does not mention her Benedictine oblature in her memoirs or in any of her extant talks or reflections. Because of the nature of those difficult Communist times, no documentation of the event has survived — neither among Hanna's personal papers (most of which were destroyed however after her death) nor in the abbey archives. We only know that the ceremony took place and that being a Benedictine oblate made a big impact on Hanna's personal life and profoundly shaped her active nursing spirituality. Information about Hanna being an oblate is based on the evidence of the surviving elderly monks living at the abbey who remember Hanna, among them Dom Leon Knabit, and from the accounts of her two Benedictine oblate friends who survived her, Wacława Bogdal and Alina Rumun, both of whom spoke and wrote about Hanna after her death, long before the cause for Hanna's canonisation was formally opened in 1998. Additionally, we know from Wacława that she was left Hanna's Benedictine oblate medal and scapular — which have survived to this day and are treasured relics.

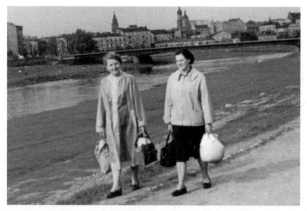

Hanna and Alina Rumun, who was also a Benedictine oblate of Tyniec Abbey. Walking along the Wisła riverbank.

It would be interesting to know if Hanna ever reflected back upon her time in New York City and her possible visits to the Cloisters Museum in Upper Manhattan, as she stood on the high cliffs by Tyniec Abbey and looked over the Wisła River onto the Kraków countryside. We cannot be sure that she was even aware of The Cloisters, although the museum was in existence when she was living at Maxwell Hall on Washington Heights, as it was officially opened in 1938. Maxwell Hall was only a ten minute bus-ride from the museum and Hanna was known to love the arts. It is hard to believe that she would not have visited the museum. In 1946 the New York museum did not look as it does today, but there was an interesting parallel between the two edifices — both perched high on river cliffs with spectacular views of the surrounding area. But whereas Tyniec Abbey is a living Benedictine monastery housed in a Romanesque building, albeit heavily reconstructed in the baroque style during the 16th and 17th centuries, and is a functioning place of prayer and scholarship, The Cloisters Museum is reconstructed from the architectural elements of several Benedictine Abbeys which had been built in the Romanesque style; namely Saint-Michel-de-Cuxa and Saint-Guilhem-le-Désert (both in the South of France), and the Church of San Martín in Fuentidueña in central Spain. It is, nevertheless, a truly unique museum. Most importantly, both places are restful, inspirational and prayerful.

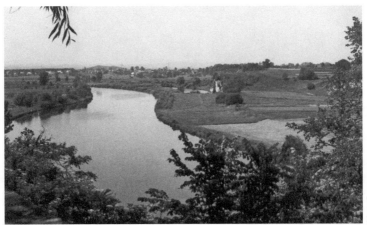

Marie Romagnano

View from Tyniec Abbey on the Wisła River

Hanna spent many summer evenings at Tyniec praying, meditating and unwinding from the pressures of her pastoral work. She would often attend the Divine Office, in which she participated with great attention, if initially somewhat passively, as the entire Liturgy of the Hours was then sung in Latin, in plainchant. Every year she joined in the prayerful, ancient liturgies of Holy Week. She would leave her home in Kraków early in Holy Week and with her fellow oblate friends and co-workers from the Parish Nursing movement — Wacława and Alina — spend the rest of Holy Week at the Abbey, only returning to her apartment on Sunday morning, after the first Mass of Easter had been celebrated at dawn. She would then burst into her apartment or friend's house with the joyful words, 'Christ is Risen! — and I am starving — what do you have to eat!? She repeated this ritual every year.

The oblates stayed in an attic, in a house close to the abbey — and as Hanna mentions in her letters, postcards and reports, they enjoyed themselves immensely. There was much laughter and many joyful memories from those days and weeks spent at the Abbey. Hanna was enthralled (as many before her and afterwards), by the writings (often no more than scribbles and notes) of past monks along the sides of ancient manuscripts and old chant books. She copied some of these comments into her own papers and often referred to them, as they greatly amused her.

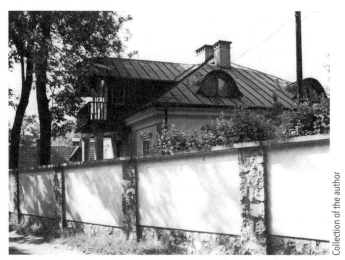

Collection of the author

Hanna and her oblate friends – Wacława Bogdal and Alina Rumun
used to stay in the attic of this house when they visited Tyniec Abbey.

After hearing the passage from the Acts of the Apostles, 'We
have likewise become servants of the royal priesthood of the whole
People of God, of all the baptized, so that we may proclaim the *'mighty
works of God'* in Latin *'magnalia Dei'*. (Acts 2:11); and also in the
Antiphon for Pentecost, '… *loquebantur variis lingus apostoli magnalia
Dei,*' ('The apostles spoke in tongues of the Greatness of God/Great
works of God'); she started using that Latin phrase with her friends.
Whenever she wanted to say that she had something important to
transmit, and wanted to change the subject, she would preface the
statement with the words, '…and now let us move onto *magnalia Dei*',
and she always had in mind the wellbeing of her patients, their welfare.
This light-hearted assimilation of liturgical phrases into her regular
vocabulary was to become characteristic of Hanna — especially after
she became an oblate and spent more time in Tyniec Abbey where she
heard these Latin expressions.

If the first pillar of Hanna's spirituality was a love for, and an
active interpretation of the gospel narratives, especially those referring
to social interactions and the healing actions of Christ, the second
pillar of Hanna's spirituality was her love for scripture-based prayer.
It is the Holy Spirit that guides the heart through meditation on the
scriptures and teaches us how 'to pray the scriptures.' Hanna took

naturally to the ancient method of Benedictine meditation — *Lectio Divina* (or holy reading) — as it echoed her natural inclination to quiet contemplative and reflective prayer, and she found much solace in its ancient richness.

Hanna was instinctively drawn to a deep and private prayer-life. Her oblate friends observed that while Hanna lived out her prayer in active nursing service to the abandoned and the poor who were sick, she often went apart to pray and meditate. Hanna did this in order to be alone, where no one would interrupt her prayer, where she could be by herself with Christ, undisturbed by the distractions of professional and social life. Hanna wrote in a letter, 'One needs to make for oneself space to think, for personal prayer apart from the psalms, even separate from the Holy Mass. Otherwise you wither like a cut reed'.

Wacława, her oblate friend, recounted that often when they were walking together in the Tatra mountains, Hanna would walk a little behind the others, or slightly detached from the group in order to be 'alone', to reflect and to pray. As has often been said, personal prayer exists at the centre of any spirituality — including nursing spirituality — and being an oblate helped Hanna to maintain a deeper prayer life, which in turn sustained her active nursing ministry.

Hanna's spirituality was shaped by her meditations on the Bible, and through her Benedictine prayer-life she deepened her understanding of other Christian texts. She started to identify more closely with a scripture-based approach to prayer, as one can see in her poetry and her statements to her nurses in the Parish movement and to nursing religious sisters. She was also clearly excited by the various conciliar and post-conciliar documents that were being published at the time and which the monks were working on — translating and editing.

She avidly read encyclicals as they came out from Rome, and the many Council documents, following closely the outcomes of various episcopal meetings and Synod pronouncements especially those concerning changes, approaches and explanations about aspects of faith, worship and the role of the laity. She was also greatly influenced by teaching of the Second Vatican Council on the mystery of the universal priesthood of the laity and the new understanding of the role of the laity in the Church. In a description of her work to nursing sisters, she referred to the pre-conciliar encyclical of Pope Pius XII — *Mystici*

Corporis Christi — written during the war, in 1943. In that document the Pope expanded upon St Paul's words in 1 Corinthians, chapter 12:

> But a body calls also for a multiplicity of members, which are linked together in such a way as to help one another. And as in the body when one member suffers, all the other members share its pain, and the healthy members come to the assistance of the ailing, so in the Church the individual members do not live for themselves alone, but also help their fellows, and all work in mutual collaboration for the common comfort and for the more perfect building up of the whole Body. (15)

Hanna took these words very much to heart and the following statement a few lines further on:

> ...the Fathers of the Church sing the praises of this Mystical Body of Christ, with its ministries, its variety of ranks, its officers, it conditions, its orders, its duties, they are thinking not only of those who have received Holy Orders, but of all those too, who, following the evangelical counsels, pass their lives... actively among men, ... also of those who, though living in the world, consecrate themselves wholeheartedly to spiritual or corporal works of mercy...(17)

Hanna followed the evangelical counsels in this way, and she became an avid reader of the later Council documents that were being translated into Polish concerning the role of the laity in the Church. These documents were being published and distributed in the 1960s at the conclusion of the Second Vatican Council. In the document *Lumen Gentium*, the Council affirmed that

> ...the faithful, in virtue of their royal priesthood, join in the offering of the Eucharist. They likewise exercise that priesthood in receiving the sacraments, in prayer and thanksgiving, in the witness of a holy life, and by self-denial and active charity. (Ch. 2. 10.101)

Hanna would often return to this mystery of universal priest-hood in her writings and talks to her Parish Nurses. It is a deep mystery of the Christian faith, which helped define and mould her active, lay, nursing spirituality. In 1970, in a talk prepared for a congress in Rome concerning lay evangelisation, (which Hanna in the end could not attend, because she was denied a visa by the Polish Communist government), she noted that the ill person is also, '…a member of the people of God, what's more they are not only an immensely important member of the Mystical Body, that they too, the same as everyone else, must participate in the universal Kingly, Prophetic and Priestly states.' For Hanna, no one was exempted from this universal truth.

She was herself empowered by the Council documents and proceeded to share her prayerful insights with her patients and nurses. Hanna had a listening, reflective Benedictine soul, and at the same time she was a beautiful example of an active lay woman, influenced and nurtured by the teachings of the Second Vatican Council. She was willing to share these fruits of the Council with everyone she encountered. She found the monks at Tyniec Abbey supportive in her quest for deeper insights into these and other conciliar statements. Hanna felt sufficiently comfortable as an oblate of Tyniec Abbey that she was able to grow and develop spiritually, in harmony with these new insights, revealed by the Holy Spirit and proclaimed to the Christian world. In Poland, these conciliar documents were promulgated by the monks of Tyniec Abbey.

In the centre of Kraków where Hanna lived and worked, one was never far from the sound of church bells calling the faithful to recite the Angelus three times a day. Hanna's post-war apartment on Łobzowska Street was situated directly across the street from a Carmelite monastery of nuns, and she was woken each morning by the tolling of the chapel bell for the recitation of the Angelus. This was repeated at midday and in the evening. Likewise, the Kraków School of Nursing on Kopernika Street, where she worked as a young nurse upon her return from France, and again much later, after the conclusion of the Second World War, is situated in an area that is surrounded by five churches and two convent chapels. Indeed, the School of Nursing where she worked for so many years is also situated opposite a Carmelite monastery of nuns, the second Carmelite monastery in the city, and thus for most of her time in Kraków, Hanna both lived and worked within the sounds of monastic church bells, which would joyfully ring out the message of the Incarnation.

Hanna, the overtly busy and bubbly nurse while all the while an interiorly contemplative Benedictine oblate, would feel drawn to prayer every time she heard the Angelus bell, and like the monks in Tyniec Abbey, she would reflect however briefly on the greatest mystery of all: on the mystery of the humanity of God.

Hanna's practical theology was always solidly grounded in her nursing practice, and it stemmed from her deep appreciation of this mystery of God Incarnate. The very last prayer that Hanna was known to meditate upon, just a few hours before her death, was the Angelus. Hanna, as a nurse, was entranced by the mystery of God becoming human and she therefore understood the value of standing beneath the Cross, while aware of the joyous implications of a new dawn — the Resurrection. Life as an oblate supported Hanna in living out more deeply these interrelated Christian truths. Finally, as Dom Leon Knabit often said about Hanna, she managed with the help of God to maintain a perfect Benedictine balance of *Ora et Labora*, of work and prayer, in her chosen way of life.

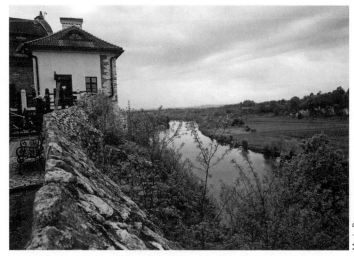

View from Tyniec Abbey

CHAPTER 11

A Restless Heart: Forced into Retirement

Let us allow God to act; He brings things to completion when we least expect it.
— St Vincent de Paul

As with many who retire early, Hanna's retirement was anything but restful or uneventful. It was simply a convenient time to change the direction of her nursing career. Initially it gave her time to finish co-authoring and editing a textbook with Kazimiera Skobyłko on nursing care in the community, which was published in 1960 under the title *Pielęgniarstwo w Otwartej Opiece Zdrowotnej* (Nursing in the Community). This book became a nursing best-seller, with several reprints and editions. The fourth and final edition was published posthumously in 1973.

Throughout her retirement, Hanna remained an active member of the Polish Nurses Association (PNA), *Polskie Towarzystwo Pielęgniarskie*, which in 1957 had been restructured to resume the work of the pre-war professional association which had been dissolved by the Germans in 1939. She was an active member of the PNA, as well as serving both on the Association's National Executive Board and on the Council of the Kraków Regional Branch, with special responsibilities for the Historical Section. The significance of these details lies in the fact that these institutions belonged to Poland's Socialist establishment. Some commentators have noted surprise that Hanna would even want to join a 'Socialist' organisation, such as the Polish Nurses Association, (PNA), but she felt that the PNA was her professional organisation, and that the best course of action was to support it and work from within its structures to achieve change, rather than boycott it for political reasons. Her presence in the organisation was a moderating influence on the brash new generation of politically-appointed leaders of the nursing profession.

As for the reinstated nursing journal, *Pielęgniarka Polska*, which she had helped to establish before the war, she carried on contributing to it from 1949 to 1958. From 1958 until 1970 she wrote for its new version, *Pielęgniarka i Położna*, which was aimed at both nurses and midwives. Finally, even the Socialist government decided it should recognise Hanna's pioneering work, and so in 1957 she was awarded a medal for exemplary activity in promoting public health nursing. Then in 1971, she was awarded the Cross of the Knights of the Order of the Rebirth of Poland, *Krzyż Kawalerski Orderu Odrodzenia Polski.*

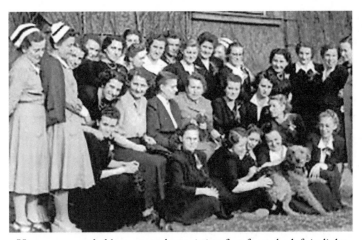

Hanna surrounded by past students sitting first from the left in light blouse. Hanna kept in touch with her nursing students; many became good friends and worked with her in the Parish Nursing project.

In 1969, with a change in government and a slight thawing of the hard-line Stalinist approach of the 1950s, although now already well into her retirement, she was called upon by the Ministry of Health to act as deputy spokesperson for Health Care Workers, attached to the regional commission for professional conduct (*Okręgowa Komisja Kontroli Zawodowej*). This involved sitting on many committees, participating in the resolution of ethical issues pertaining to the nursing profession and hearing professional conduct cases. Sitting on the hearings pained Hanna as she listened to countless examples of poor conduct and bad patient care. Given that Hanna was known to oppose the prevailing Socialist ideologies imposed on all professionals at that time, this exceptional move by the authorities, to appoint Hanna to the conduct commission, points to the high esteem in which she was regarded even by the socialists — at a local if not national level.

It could be argued of course that she was a token representative on the government committees — a single high-profile non-governmental voice. However, those who knew Hanna well were quick to point out her intelligence, professional integrity and unfailing concern for the good of nurses. It is more likely that she was, however unorthodox from a political perspective, simply an outstanding example of a professional nurse. She could be counted upon to be discreet; and she was a pleasure to work with, an obvious asset to any working party. Even though Hanna was not a member of the Communist Party, and was not a Socialist, and had other political 'points' against her, such as coming from the landed gentry and the bourgeoisie, and being a practising Catholic and having suspicious contacts with people abroad — despite all these so-called 'disadvantages', the Ministry of Health nonetheless conceded that she was dependable, fair and without personal axes to grind. In other words, Hanna was very experienced, and gifted with diplomacy and tact. There is evidence that Hanna seized this opportunity to bring to governmental proceedings and professional conduct meetings a refreshing *non-socialist* approach to problem-solving.

She astutely observed a few years later in her memoirs that removing individuals from pedestals may sometimes be necessary in order to correctly reinterpret history, but this should only be done if the intention is to provide a more truthful picture of reality; it should never be done in malice. She concludes, '…we must never forget that a person's ethical norm is always his or her conscience, which of course does not negate objective norms…', a statement which is still very topical today. And so it was that 'the system' would honour her at times, and at others would take away her livelihood and consider her a political embarrassment. But for Hanna, the only true measure of a person's integrity was an ethically sensitive conscience. As Kipling noted in his classic poem, '…if you can meet with Triumph and Disaster and treat these two imposters just the same…' you have achieved much. Hanna demonstrated throughout her life how she could negotiate her way between these two imposters, especially during the Communist era.

At the same time that Hanna received her awards, similar official recognition by the Socialist state had been bestowed on her friend Aleksandra Dąmbska and Jadwiga Romanowska, one of Hanna's oldest nursing-school friends from the WSN and subsequently a good colleague. Both Aleksandra and Jadwiga were living and working at that time in Gdańsk, in the north of Poland by the Baltic Sea. Aleksandra had been relocated to Gdańsk from her town of Lwów in Southeastern Poland after the war, since her own home town was now within the borders of the Ukraine. As was the case with Hanna, the State's recognition of their work did not stop the Socialist authorities from dismissing them from their nursing positions a few months later. They too were considered to be a dangerous influence on student nurses. Jadwiga Romanowska had been dismissed as director of the Gdańsk School of Nursing, together with most of her staff, including Aleksandra.

Upon losing her job in Gdańsk, Aleksandra decided to retire and go to live in Kraków with her sister, Izydora Dąmbska, a well-known professor of analytical philosophy, at that time working at the Jagiellonian University. Dr Dąmbska lived in a fairly large apartment in the centre of the old city, and conducted seminars from her home, which many aspiring young intellectuals would attend — including the young Fr Karol Wojtyła.

By moving to Kraków, Aleksandra became unexpectedly available to help Hanna in the Parish Nursing Project. There is no doubt that Aleksandra was a great asset to Hanna in executing this parish-based project. Aleksandra's young relatives remember the flurry of activity that pervaded the apartment prior to every retreat in Trzebinia, since the sisters also had a telephone (essential to coordinate the project), and since the apartment was located across the road from the main university buildings and St Anne's Church, it was easy to get hold of student volunteers. Like Hanna, Aleksandra was an exceptionally good and religiously-motivated nurse. When she died, the Capuchin priest hurrying through the church on Loretańska Street, to console the bereaved family waiting outside, kept repeating 'She was a saint, she was a saint....'

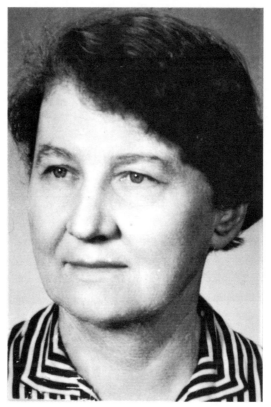

Hanna in the 1950s

CHAPTER 12

Helping Christ to Carry His Cross: Parish Nursing
1956-1973

The most beautiful and stirring adventure that can happen to
you is the personal meeting with Jesus.
— St Pope John Paul II

Hanna was no longer an employee of the regional health department or the school of nursing and the fate of the chronically ill was no longer her official business. However, there were still sick and housebound individuals. Hanna was convinced that something had to done for these people and this neglected area of community nursing had to be addressed. Although retired, Hanna was still a qualified nurse, and so she was often asked to help with the nursing care of relatives, friends and acquaintances. Through this unofficial work she was constantly reminded of the dismal state of affairs that prevailed in the field of community nursing.

After the war, the Polish healthcare system did not include provision for what is now called community or district nursing. While there was reasonable acute healthcare provision, organised in the style of Soviet medicine, and a widespread system across the country of outpatient community clinics, there was no established care for people who were housebound, whether chronically ill or disabled or recovering from an episode of acute sickness. When Hanna still had responsibility for training student nurses on their community placements, she would take them to visit the housebound and chronically sick and through this educational route, community patients would be given appropriate care and nursing support. This was the case in Kraków, but not all schools of nursing in the country had sessions on community nursing care and often there was no provision made in the curriculum for community nursing studies, so no student community placements were arranged. A generation of nurses was being trained that had no idea about the needs of patients outside a hospital, living in the community. Now that Hanna was retired, these community visits which she once used to arrange and supervise for her students, were not taking place in Kraków either.

Upon returning from the USA, in the early fifties, while still teaching at the school of nursing, she had tried to interest several religious congregations of nursing sisters in Kraków to work with her in setting up a parish-based district nursing project. She even ran a few community nursing training sessions for the sisters who already had nursing qualifications.

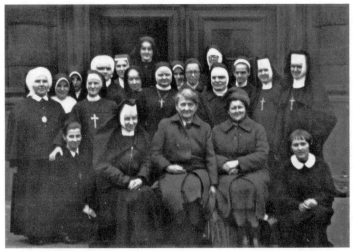

Hanna in the centre with Alina Rumun on her right and Sister Serafina Palushek on her left, at the conclusion of a course in community nursing for religious sisters.

But the political and social climate in the country now made this project impossible. The sisters declined to help, fearful about their own precarious legal status. Additionally, the Communist authorities refused to allow religious sisters to study in state-run nursing schools. Consequently, the sisters had already begun to change their focus from healthcare to other areas of pastoral work. There were now insufficient sisters left with relevant nursing qualifications.

The only nursing work the sisters could legitimately undertake at that time was the institutional care of severely handicapped children, and the care of vulnerable, chronically ill and severely disabled adults, including those with psychiatric disorders. Care was delivered in huge institutions, and these were usually situated well out of town. The Communist authorities argued that in undertaking nursing and social work in areas where there was a chronic shortage of qualified help, due to the difficult nature of work, the sisters would be doing a job that had to be done and they would be at the same time kept out of sight. In the process, the authorities unwittingly helped to preserve a modicum of dignity and compassionate care for the most marginalised in society, by assigning their care to dedicated nursing religious.

Out of the socio-political chaos of those times, a few fine examples of cooperation between Church, and community and health services continued to flourish, albeit accidentally and, as far as the Communist authorities were concerned, unintentionally. Not even the Daughters of Charity, who had run hospitals before the war and still had many relatively young qualified nursing sisters, could help Hanna. In 1953/54, Hanna went with her oblate friend Wacława Bogdal to the assistant Bishop of Kraków, Fr Jopa, to seek his advice on the matter, but the time was not right. Since there were no religious nursing sisters who could help with the project, little progress was made at that time.

Meanwhile, as Hanna noted in her memoirs, the years 1956 and 1957 were inordinately difficult for her. However, she was undaunted and, after much reflection and prayer, decided that if the sisters could not help her to set up and run the community nursing project, the only option was to try to structure it as a bottom-up, lay-led initiative, based on the zeal and efforts of committed and qualified members of the laity, preferably with the support of the Church. In June 1957, Zofia Szlendak, a friend and Kraków-based community nursing colleague, advised Hanna that for this type of pastoral problem she needed to approach *Wujek* (Uncle) for some wise counsel. This was no sooner proposed than it was done.

Wujek turned out to be a young assistant priest at St Florian's Church in the centre of Kraków, Fr Karol Wojtyła. Father Wojtyła was already well known in Kraków, since he was also engaged in teaching

activities and pastoral work among academics and students; it is the
students who had named him *Wujek* as a form of protection and cover
from prying Communist authorities.

Writing about that first meeting with Fr Wojtyła, Hanna says
that she was immediately struck by his ability to focus and to listen.
He was, she noted, '...all attention and all ears!' Father Karol told
her to come back in a few days' time while he thought the problem
through and looked around for sources of help. Several days later, Fr
Karol invited the nurses to meet with him and Fr Ferdinand Machay,
the parish priest and canon of the medieval Basilica of the Blessed
Virgin Mary, (known locally as The Mariacki Church) situated in the
old town square.

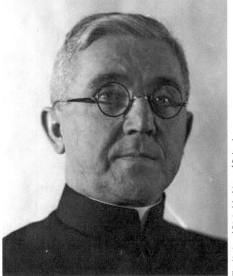

Fr Ferdinand Machay, who helped Hanna to
start the Parish Nursing movement in his parish.

Father Machay (1889-1967) was an interesting person and
certainly not a typical parish priest. He is the subject of several fascinating biographies, and even during his lifetime he was something
of a legend. Above all, Fr Machay was an intelligent, holy priest, a
patriot and socially active. Hanna knew of his work and reputation
from her wartime activities in Kraków, when their paths had crossed

in connection with organising help for refugees and placing children and Jews in safe home.

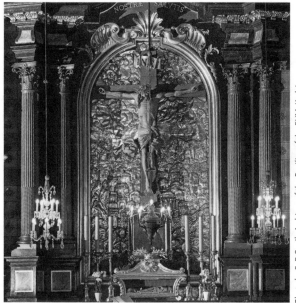

Hanna prayed with Fr Karol Wojtyla in front of this miraculous Crucifix in the Basilica of the BVM, Kraków, for the approval of Parish Nursing by Fr Ferdinand Machay.

Sure of her purpose, but with trepidation, and after praying before the miraculous medieval crucifix in the Mariacki Church, Hanna explained her idea to him, adding that she already knew who could and would help her in the elaborate scheme of parish-based nursing. She had in mind a lay-based movement consisting of committed volunteers. As Hanna later recalled in her memoirs, 'I was immediately struck by his simplicity and wisdom'. Father Machay at once agreed to help Hanna, characteristically adding, to Hanna's delight, '…only remember, I don't want to have any trouble from you! You're the expert, not me.'

Pope St John Paul II (Karol Wojtyła) in his memoirs (*Rise, let us be on our way*), states that he came to know Hanna through Fr Machay and that 'thanks to the efforts of Hanna Chrzanowska, the apostolate among the sick emerged and started to take shape in the archdiocese'.

Hanna was to work closely with Fr Machay over the next few years and received much support from him. Shortly before his death, he said that his involvement with Hanna and the parish nursing project was the highlight of his pastoral endeavours. Meanwhile, with the passage of time, Hanna started to familiarise herself with the work and activities of Fr Karol Wojtyła, and eventually, the pair were to become an effective pastoral team.

Once again, Hanna considered asking the religious of Kraków to help her establish her new project. She approached the Sisters of the Holy Soul of Christ, a medieval nursing order, which, before the war, ran hospitals in central Europe, not only in Poland. But the sister who was sent to help Hanna was called away to another assignment after only a few weeks.

The first months of work on the parish nursing project were extremely hard. Hanna had only the help of Alina Rumun, and then only part-time. Alina was working full-time at the hospital and spent all her spare time with Hanna on the community project. Hanna became so busy looking after patients, and had so many requests for help that she became overwhelmed with the workload. At that point Archbishop Baziak (1890–1962), invited her to his office and told her to approach the Congregation of the Sisters of St Joseph, who had recently arrived in Kraków at his request, and who were looking for an apostolate. Moreover, Archbishop Baziak personally instructed the Sisters of St Joseph to cooperate with Hanna; and from that time onwards the work-load became easier. Hanna found the Sisters of St Joseph responsive to her nursing ideology, and she noted in her memoirs that from her first meeting with them, in their small cosy parlour, she knew that they could and would work well together.

Hanna writes that she was so full of gratitude and relief that a source of permanent help was found for the work that, as soon as the meeting was over, she hurried to Smoleńska Street — to the chapel of the Sisters of St Felix (the Felician Sisters), where there was exposition of the Blessed Sacrament. She intended to thank God for the successful outcome of the meeting. But it was late, and the doors to the sisters' chapel were already closed for the night. Hanna relates in her memoirs how she simply fell to her knees on the pavement, outside the convent walls, and prayed.

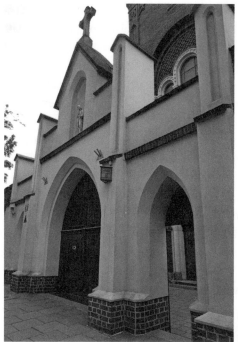

Doors to the Sisters of St Felix convent, where there was perpetual
exposition of the Blessed Sacrament. Smoleńska Street, Kraków.

This account is fascinating, for it illustrates several important
points about Hanna's spirituality at this time. Firstly, it demonstrates
her profound belief in the presence of Christ in the Blessed Sacrament, and it displays her genuine and uncomplicated response to this
faith. Of course, she could have quietly prayed without kneeling on the
pavement outside the convent doors, but she *chose* to fall on her knees.
The presence of two sets of heavy wooden doors could not separate her
from the presence of Christ her Lord, located in the chapel beyond.

Hanna's simple faith in this instance is awe-inspiring, and the
way she responded was uniquely hers. One might argue that the very
fact that she mentioned this incident in her memoirs suggests that
this impulsive behaviour was unusual, even for her. But it was not
completely out of character. Hanna often prayed in that chapel and
she knew that there was exposition of the Blessed Sacrament in the
chapel. Going to the chapel to say 'Thank you,' was the first thing that
came to mind.

For Hanna to pray openly, on the pavement outside the closed convent doors in Communist Poland of the mid-1950s also speaks volumes about Hanna's impulsive and endearing rashness. If this was Hanna acting spontaneously and typically, one can begin to appreciate the superhuman efforts that she made in order to conceal her clandestine wartime activities. She must have exercised extraordinary patience and self-control in order to accomplish the seemingly impossible during the war years. This spontaneous behaviour, which reflected her vibrant spiritual life, demonstrates that she enjoyed God's ever-present support and protection.

In the autumn of 1957, after her meeting with Fr Machay, the Kraków-based Catholic weekly newspaper, *Tygodnik Powszechny*, published an article written by Hanna entitled *Świat nie jest pusty* (The world is not empty), in which she explained the plight of the chronically ill in Kraków and their lack of nursing services. The article was greeted with such enthusiasm by the people of Kraków that many nurses immediately volunteered to work with Hanna. Donations began to pour into the editorial offices. Hanna used this money to buy initial medical supplies and equipment.

Hanna continued to receive support for her parish project from her old nursing friends, colleagues, and former students from the Kraków School of Nursing — people such as Alina and Wacława Bogdal, both of whom, like Hanna, were also Benedictine oblates. Alina was to become Hanna's assistant and upon Hanna's death she continued the parish nursing project. In 2007 shortly before her death, Alina received the Florence Nightingale Medal from the International Red Cross for her services to community parish nursing — an honour which she often said was really intended for Hanna. During Hanna's lifetime the Polish Communist government did not allow nurses to be put forward for this prestigious international award.

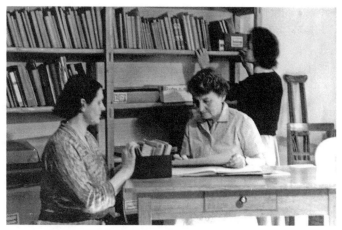

Alina Rumun helping Hanna with some patient notes in
Fr Machay's presbytery.

As already noted, Hanna also received nursing help from Aleksandra Dąmbska, her old friend who was forced to retire from teaching nurses in Gdańsk, for political reasons. She joined Hanna's parish nursing project a little later, and was to be closely involved with the project until a few years before her death in 1988.

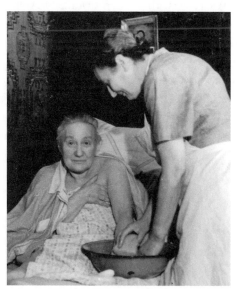

Aleksandra Dąmbska washing Mme Cecilia – a bed-bound patient.

Gradually, various nursing sisterhoods joined Hanna's work, especially the Franciscan sisters from the Congregation of St. Felix, known in the USA and Canada as Felician sisters — in front of whose chapel Hanna had fallen to her knees — and the Sisters of The Sacred Heart, who worked in the Bishop's palace and were specifically sent to help Hanna by the new bishop of Kraków, Karol Wojtyła. Eventually, the Daughters of Charity of St Vincent de Paul were also able to provide her with young nursing sisters. Additionally, Hanna received support from seminarians who were studying in Kraków, since the town hosted three diocesan seminaries, several congregations of friars and priests that had noviciates, and two orders of nursing brothers.

To Hanna, Alina, Wacława and Aleksandra and other qualified nurses fell the task of coordinating the delivery of care, which various non-nurse volunteers were taught to provide. Hanna noted that at one point over a hundred volunteers were involved. She also organised training sessions and preparatory nursing classes for helpers who had a minimum of nursing experience, as well as gave separate lessons in community care to the sisters and nurses who only had nursing experience from working in hospitals — which was most of them. Finally Hanna, motivated both the students and the teaching academic community to join the project. The students worked as volunteers, providing ongoing social support to the many housebound and chronically ill patients. Without the help and enthusiasm of these students, it would have been very difficult, if not impossible, to run many of the projects.

One engineering student — Jerzy Ciesielski, a member of the Focolare Movement, and a good friend of Fr Karol Wojtyła, took on the role of coordinator of the students' involvement and after his tragic premature death in 1970, his wife Danuta assumed this role.

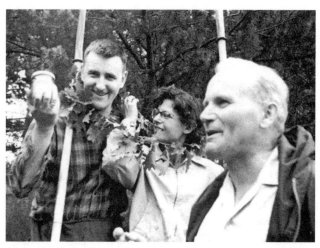

Venerable Jerzy Ciesielski with his wife Danuta and the young
Father Karol Wojtyla.

Today the Church in Kraków considers Venerable Servant of
God Jerzy Ciesielski, like Hanna, to be a candidate for sainthood. All
over Kraków, from all walks of life, people contributed in whatever
way they could, towards the parish nursing project.

The public's eagerness to help Hanna was partly the result of her
charismatic talks to members of religious orders, church congregations,
clergy, deanery meetings, at retreat centres, to students in schools of
nursing, and to academic gatherings in universities. Without the help
of this vast army of volunteers the project would never have taken off
to the extent that it did. However, Hanna was always keen to point
out that the help of volunteers and the work of her parish nurses and
the visits by parish workers to the housebound and infirm were never
intended to hamper, alter, or negate the necessity for the natural relationships between individuals and within families.

Hanna was quite clear that the project was not intended solely to
provide company for lonely and isolated parishioners; the nurses were
to go to homes where there was a clear nursing need. If parishioners
required other types of intervention, these could hopefully be arranged
with her army of volunteers but, her community nurses were not to be
distracted from their primary objective which was the nursing care of
chronically or seriously ill individuals, in their own homes. If people

were already in the habit of dropping in on their elderly neighbours, this was to be supported and encouraged. She wrote: 'it is not our intention to remove from families and wider circles of acquaintances responsibility for the love of one's neighbour.'

The parish nurses worked to a set of rules and had a binding code of conduct which had been drawn up by Hanna together with her nurses. In 1960, this code of conduct for parish nurses was formally approved by a committee consisting of Hanna, Teresa Strzembosz, Aniela Łossow (a nursing colleague of Teresa Strzembosz from Warsaw), and Bishop Bronisław Dąbrowski, representing the Polish episcopate, and a few others. The aims of the project made it clear that parish nurses were to give priority care to the elderly infirm and chronically ill, regardless of a patient's ability to pay. The professional nurses were to be paid employees of the parish. Hanna was adamant that, provided the frail patients had a definable nursing need, parish nurses ought to go to those people. Since the parish nurses were to be qualified nurses, working for a particular parish or group of parishes, and since they were to be salaried, it was their professional duty to care for all chronically sick patients in that parish, whether they were rich or poor, educated or from a working-class background.

Hanna's revolutionary ideas concerning parish nursing were expertly put into practice over half a century before the introduction of parish nursing concepts into mainstream community nursing elsewhere. As envisaged and implemented by Hanna, parish nursing was already a realistic project well before the idea took hold in other countries. Her particular interpretation of community and faith-based nursing activities pre-dated American parish nursing programmes, and when allowance is made for the social and economic hardships imposed by the Communist authorities of that time, the professional nature of the undertaking becomes awe-inspiring.

Hanna ran into many problems with the Communist authorities, who considered her work to be ideologically subversive. Surprisingly, there were also problems from some of the religious orders, who would have preferred to see the care given to the frail elderly and chronically ill in more traditional institutional surroundings where, no doubt, they would have had more control over how the care was administered, instead of having to look after patients in their own homes. Unfortunately, power struggles, insecurity and lack of vision are not restricted to the political arena. It is all the more remarkable that Hanna managed to convince so many people of the appropriateness of her approach to the care of these individuals in the community, especially in the context of a Socialist system which thrived on, and almost exclusively approved of, institutional care.

Hanna continued to write for nurses, but now almost exclusively for her parish nurses. She wrote for them a perceptive tract, *An Examination of a Nurse's Conscience*, and a leaflet on *Ethical Issues in Nursing Practice*. Hanna's nurses and co-workers greatly appreciated her caring attitude and concern for their welfare, as well as her ongoing hands-on participation in the parish nursing project. Nurses felt comfortable in her company, and those closest to her affectionately called her *Cioteczka* (Auntie), a title which amused Hanna and which she used herself in turn, when communicating with them.

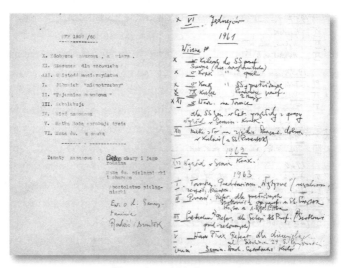

Hanna's scribbled notes

The parish nursing project was never intended as a form of volunteer work for qualified community nurses, although its success relied on the goodwill and cooperation of unpaid volunteers. The volunteers were trained and coordinated by paid professional parish nurses. Parish nursing was an unusual phenomenon in Poland during the 1960s and 1970s, one which was not well understood even by parish priests. Initially, the priests tended to treat the parish nursing project as an extension of the parish's existing pastoral response to the needy in the area, albeit conducted by 'good Catholic nurses.' Another problem with the prevailing attitude of parish priests was their reaction of negation and disbelief that chronically ill people might be living in their parishes. They claimed to know everyone in their parishes and that there were no housebound patients or sick people languishing in garrets and basements. But this view was to change with time.

Hanna wrote a series of reflections about several of her significant parish nursing experiences. The case studies were written in the form of vignettes, describing in sensitive but also amusing fashion some of the more memorable ones, to convey to others what the work entailed. It is clear from these case studies that Hanna genuinely enjoyed being with her patients, she cared deeply for them, wished them well and accepted them exactly as they were, which is why she was fond of them and could laugh and cry with them. She said in a presentation to a group of Daughters of Charity, 'For many years I have been a nursing instructor, then a principal of a school of nursing. I was a manager, a director, and an examiner. Therefore, what joy it is at last, in my old age, to get my hands on the sick: to wash them, scrub them. Flick off their fleas. It's the nature of these basic, fundamental procedures — which are most important to the them. So restrain your egos, and let yourself go onto the wide waters of Love; not with clenched teeth, and not for some sort of thought about mortification, and not because you are forced to do so, and certainly not treating the ill patient as some sort of 'ladder to heaven'. Only when we can really let go of ourselves, and our prejudices can we trully serve Christ in the sick.'

Writing for a Kraków newspaper, she described some typical cases that parish nurses were involved with, so that the readers — who were potential financial supporters of the project or even future volunteers in the movement — could gain some understanding of the nature of the work. She wrote that '...there was an elderly woman with a massive brain tumour spreading down to her eyebrows. She was unimaginably filthy, with bedsores. Her help at home consisted of a psychopathic daughter who worked eight hours a day outside of the home, and a second daughter who was schizophrenic and requiring help herself — but who was outside the psychiatric care system. The toenails and fingernails of the ill woman were so long and so thick that you could hear them drop to the floor with a thud, as we cut them. When we turned the woman over, she would try to pinch us and she howled in pain ...meanwhile fleas dropped off her like so many grains of sands, while her wounds were infested with them, under a layer of dirt and creams. The nurses managed to find her after several years of abandoned neglect, barely a week before the death. But her spirits were up, she was totally lucid and she was content now that she was washed and being nursed. At least she died with some semblance of being finally cared for.'

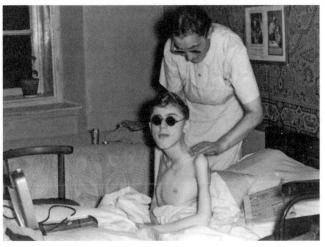

Parish Nursing

In another example, Hanna's nurses looked after a woman whose drunken husband had thrown her out of a second-floor flat where she fortunately landed in a pile of snow. But she broke both her legs and her back. In another case a woman who was incurably ill was laid up in bed and unable to move, awaiting death. Her husband could not wait for her to die, while her sons called her vile names and mistreated her. She suffered greatly from the psychological pain of abandonment and ridicule from her own family. Her death was a release from all her suffering. But some cases were more upliftling, even sometimes amusing. In one case that Hanna was personally involved with, an elderly frail man was tenderly looking after his even more frail convalescing wife. The elderly gentleman who wore dark glasses and was almost blind, was also unsteady on his feet. One day as he started chatting about the meaning of someone's name, Hanna suddenly realised that he had been one of her professors in high school — and who even then wore dark glasses. 'How could I not have recognised you?' she asked him. Some time later he said to her, 'You know what was so lovely about you, when you recognised me — it was the way you immediately got up from your chair — just as in the old days at school.'

Hanna not only took care of the elderly housebound in need of nursing care, she also tried to reach out to the handicapped young-sters who had been shut away in homes and flats, sometimes for years on end, usually unschooled and all of them ignored by the state authorities. One such young girl was Elżbieta (Ela) Łubinska, who was initially extremely sceptical that anyone would want to visit her, especially another young person such as a student, and give her lessons. In fact, in time, she responded so well to visits and tutorials, which were delivered by university students, that she was persuaded in spite of being wheelchair-bound to attend a regular high school, where she caught up with her schooling and eventually attended university — and all because of Hanna's determination. As Ela used to say, to anyone willing to listen, Hanna would not take no for an answer. Ela became a great admirer of Hanna and a faithful friend.

Such an open attitude to those in need confirms Hanna's expan-sive and uncomplicated approach to others. It proves her enormous personal and emotional investment in others. She experienced to the full the true significance of 'the other'. For Hanna the sick and infirm *Other* person was to be unconditionally accepted and seen in the light of faith, as Christ himself.

All of Hanna's nursing life, she tried to acknowledge the human-ity which she shared with the patients that she nursed. She eventually managed not only to empathise with them but to recognise her own life's meaning through the care that she delivered. Hanna received life and energy from her patients, and in them she encountered God. This mutual exchange of grace enriched both parties.

In December 1968, Hanna was asked to deliver a short account of her Parish Nursing work in The Mariacki Basilica, in Kraków's old town square. The talk was very short, of approximately thirty-two typewritten lines, and she proceeded to explain to the congregation not only the connection between the Basilica, Fr Ferdinand Machay (at that time, just recently deceased), and the foundations of Parish Nursing, but actually to give some insight as to why she saw the mystery of Our Lady of the Visitation as such an appropriate model for Catholic community nurses. She explained why she chose Our Lady, who hastened to visit her elderly pregnant cousin as a role model, and how Mary's neighbourly gesture inspired her work. She pointed out that Fr Machay and herself had originally met to discuss the project in the Basilica itself, praying first for a few minutes in front of the medieval altar of Christ Crucified before they proceeded together to the presbytery.

She commented that because she and Fr Machay started their discussions concerning the nursing project at the foot of the cross, in the company of Mary, the project was assured of divine help. Hanna said she believed that since Mary accompanied the project from the start, then she was also with all the nurses, the shut-ins, and the elderly patients whom they cared for. Mary would continue to be involved in the project. Hanna concluded her short presentation with a little prayer into which she wove the gospel narrative of Mary leaving in haste (Lk 1:39), and concluded with disarming womanly sincerity, since '…We are accompanied by the Servant of the Lord, who is running in great haste to help the needy, joyfully singing, attuned to the voice of Her Son, and later standing under the Cross… Therefore, [may She] plead forgiveness on our behalf; [O, Mary], even when we in our lowliness do not manage to run to help others with haste like yours — traversing over the hills — ask nonetheless, without delay, for mercy to be speedily given to us…'

Hanna believed that her nurses brought the presence of Christ, to the frail and ill and disheartened — to the sick. She added that the greatest joy and mystery of nursing was that not only do nurses serve Christ in their patients but that in the course of their nursing work they both represent and manifest Christ. Christ is both the wounded sufferer and the one who binds their wounds. Christ the compassionate healer was close to Hanna, and she reminded God, at least once, publicly, that her patients were the same as those whom His son so willingly healed in Judea, '…the same as those that the loving hand of your Son touched; the blind, deaf, paralysed, lame, bleeding…'

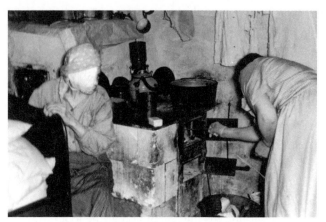

Alina Rumun nursing a patient with cancer.

Hanna worked with the marginalised and abandoned and the sick in response to the model offered by Jesus in the gospels. She wrote, ' From the very begining we tried to base our work on the gospels, where there is so much emphasis on Christ's attitude towards the sick... By our very presence we too are fulfilling an apostolic role without the use of many words... We are simply witnessing to Christ.' Through her life's work Hanna witnessed to Christ and she tried to help Him in any and every way she could: when He was ill, naked, hungry, or in prison, and she encouraged others to join her. As she said, 'Christ has given us a new commandment, illustrating it with the example of the Good Samaritan. If we are following that example, is it even right that people should have pity on us [saying that we are doing such hard work]?' In 1964, in a presentation aimed at parish workers in Warsaw, answering the question, 'Why is it that parishes are concerned with the plight of the sick and the Church has always been engaged with the care of the sick?', she replied : ' This is a direct consequence of responding to the wishes of God, as expressed in the Gospels'.

Hanna was one of the first people in Poland to promote and organise the celebration of Mass in patients' homes. For Hanna this was not to be a quick, undignified event, but a sacred occasion, 'allowing' Christ to enter the homes of the sick — and which, therefore, needed to be properly prepared and carried out. Most importantly, she wanted the sick person and their family to understand the liturgy in its post-conciliar form and to take an active part in the Mass, as was advocated in the Council documents. In this approach to religious practices Hanna here shares her reflections on the post-conciliar liturgical rite — transmitting a quiet but powerful catechesis to her patients and nurses.

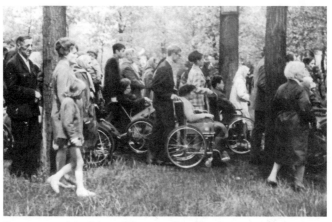

Procession of the Blessed Sacrament in Trzebinia – note the young volunteers pushing the wheelchairs. The housebound patients said that the blessing of the sick with the monstrance (as in Lourdes) was the highlight of their retreat in Trzebinia.

She knew that for patients to be able to literally invite Christ into their homes was a moving and powerful occasion, and patients were often quite emotional about the event, but for Hanna the real importance was to facilitate for her patients a fuller sharing in the Eucharist, which for many of them was a rare event, since many of them had been unable to attend Mass for a very long time. She advocated the celebration of Mass in patients' homes, because she rightfully assessed that taking them out of their apartments, in wheelchairs, to a attend Mass in their parish church, which they had been unable to do for many years, would be a disorienting and stressful experience for many of the patients. They would worry about access to toilets, drinking water or become increasingly uncomfortable in their wheelchairs.

In 1970, Hanna wrote in a paper on lay apostolates that when the sick are taken from their rooms to the parish church, if this rarely happens, then the very fact that the chronically ill person is taken out of their normal environment can provoke sufficient stress to cause at best total distraction and at worst discomfort. Often it creates a painful experience, both physically and spiritually. She wrote, 'let the ill person feel they are part of a prayerful community of faith, hope and love.' She knew this would best be achieved if the celebration of Mass was provided in the patient's own home; but always, wherever possible, with the wider family and neighbours also present. For Hanna, the celebration of Mass binds different people together and is not to be treated as a reward reserved for the select few.

Hanna was constantly harassed by the authorities for organising meetings and conferences related to her work. The Socialist authorities had made it illegal to hold unauthorised gatherings, and Hanna's work was never officially recognised, although the state was well aware of her activities. Therefore much of her educational and pastoral training of the helpers and volunteers, and many of the promotional lectures about her activities, had to take place undercover. Thus, a Day of Prayer with qualified nurses would be called 'a study day for community nurses', while study days on parish nursing were conducted in a holiday camp as part of the ongoing activities of a legitimate sports club.

This secretive approach to nurse education and the moral and spiritual development of her volunteers was not unique to Hanna and her work or, indeed, to Socialist Poland. Similar clandestine activities by church and community leaders took place throughout Communist central Europe at that time.

It is hard for us to appreciate what it was like to live under a totalitarian, socialist, anti-religious regime. Additionally, because of constant pressure from the authorities, the location of meetings had to be frequently changed, and Hanna often had to answer for her activities before the local authorities. Present at almost all her meetings was the ubiquitous Communist spy, ready to report back to the authorities on Hanna's activities. Although Hanna eventually managed to set up highly successful retreats and vacations for her housebound patients, this was prohibited in Warsaw and a retreat set up by Teresa Strzembosz was violently cut short by the secret police and army, with

the volunteers and patients unceremoniously sent home. Hanna's successes have to be seen against a background of constant uncertainty
and surveillance. Hanna managed to achieve much more than others
such as Teresa Strzembosz, who did similar work; no doubt Hanna's
tact, diplomacy and straightforward manner had much to do with this
and, at a deeper level her dependence on God.

It was not only Hanna who had to be careful how she went
about her work: all the parish nurses had to be politically astute and
aware. Sister Serafina Paluszek, a young Felician sister at the time, and
still alive today, who was delegated by her order to work with Hanna,
recounts how one day she went on her regular visit to a bed-bound
elderly man, who lived in St Florian's parish. When she entered his
room she saw that during the night he had fallen on the floor and that
she was unable to lift him onto his bed on her own. She had no one to
call upon for help, but remembered to ask herself, 'What would Hanna
do in such a situation?' At once she remembered that across the street
were soldiers' barracks, and therefore potentially, several able-bodied
lads who could help her. But they were soldiers and this was Communist Poland which proclaimed atheism and was fighting the Church
and she was a young nursing sister wearing the full habit…

She approached the duty soldier at the barrack gates and
explained her predicament. The soldier on guard was unimpressed
with her tale, but dutifully disappeared inside. After a very long time
he reappeared with another soldier behind him. Together the two soldiers returned to the fourth-floor room — but when the duty soldier
saw the condition of the patient's room he stood in the doorway in
amazement and horror. He probably had never seen such squalor and
destitution in his life. Following her directions the soldiers lifted the
man gently onto his bed. 'Do you come here often?' the duty soldier
asked her, 'Every day,' she replied. He stood and watched in awe as she
tended the man, washing him and looking after his sores. This was
most probably the first time that the soldier had witnessed the Church
in action helping the sick and vulnerable; a very different image to the
propaganda to which he had been exposed by the Communist party.
Finally he said to her, 'If you ever need help from us again, please don't
hesitate to call on us'. While the sister noted that there was no need
to lift the patient from the floor again, she did ask the soldiers if they

would help her chop some wood for his stove — and she recalled how from then onwards, every time she passed the barracks, the soldiers saluted her.

Because Parish Nursing was so new, Hanna often led the days of prayer for her volunteers herself, or she would meticulously instruct priests (when they were present) in what they were to say. She would often write out entire talks for them to give on the spirituality of suffering and the sacred vocation of healthcare workers. Unfortunately, few of Hanna's talks have survived. We only know a little about their content because the nurses and volunteers wrote down notes for themselves based on her talks and would later talk about the content of their meetings. The Secret Police who were always present, also wrote down what was being said and reported back to their officers. Their notes must have made interesting reading back in the office.

Hanna's approach to the pastoral role of the clergy, did not diminish her respect for priests and she always emphasised the special role that nurses had in preparing a patient to accept a priest into their homes. A few months before her death, she said 'We prepare the way for the priest. We must never forget that it is we who are paving the way for the work of the priest...' Hanna often said that while it was good to pray for those who were estranged from the Church, one needed to be patient concerning their readiness to ask for a priest and become reconciled with the Church. But when they agreed to receive the sacraments and died reconciled with God, Hanna was very happy, as she wrote in a letter to Cardinal Wojtyła in 1968. She made a point of writing to him about her "successes", because she realised that the Cardinal was going through a difficult time, and she wanted to cheer him up. "I want to share with Reverend Father a great joy: three of our lost sheep are no longer lost — and they were such difficult cases… I am so extremely happy and I don't know how to even start to thank God. It's such a joy, prize, and confirmation of the obvious, that our way, is the Way…" To which the Cardinal responded "…I am happy for you and all the nurses. It is so clear how pastoral is your nursing work."

Hanna had control not only over the content of the meetings which she conducted for her nurses; she also taught priests about these new methods of pastoral work, while taking care not to shock or upset her volunteers, some of whom, in the traditional fashion of the times, expected days of prayer and reflection to be led by priests. As a laywoman Hanna's innovative approach was quite unusual. This was several years before the resolutions of the Second Vatican Council concerning the increased role of the laity in Church life were widely publicised in Poland. Almost all the leading pastoral workers in Kraków eventually participated with Hanna in running Days of Prayer and conducting retreats for nurses and volunteers. Among the many priests with whom Hanna worked with closely at that time was Dom Leon Knabit OSB, now in his nineties but then a young Benedictine monk from Tyniec Abbey. He still writes and lectures, and willingly talks about Hanna, her work and her spirituality to anyone who will listen. He is in no doubt as to the extraordinary nature of the nursing spirituality which Hanna embodied.

She would often repeat that one should not force a person to pray, or to accept the sacraments, or even to be reconciled with God and the Church, but this did not preclude praying for the patient. 'Above all', she said, 'we have to be humble... we must never lord it over our patients, we should only serve them... Otherwise we would not be following the example set by Christ. Anyway, it is the ill who so often raise us up and enrich us... In comparison with such people we are simply useless servants.'

Shortly before her death, Hanna confirmed this strongly held belief, writing movingly about an incident which she had witnessed in a hospital as a young nurse many years before: 'I was working then in a hospital and I overheard a conversation between two patients where one of the patients said to the other,' "I cannot recite the *Our Father* or the *Hail Mary* anymore, I can only manage to say, 'My God', and I trust the Lord understands such abbreviations." I will never forget what he said'. Hanna knew that in order to appoach God, there is no need for many words; all that is required is an open heart focused on Christ. The people with whom she worked often reminded her of this truth.

Hanna's unique spirituality was a natural consequence of her nursing work — that is, of coming into contact with human suffering in people's homes and in hospitals — and that is why it can truly be called a nursing spirituality. She admitted in her memoirs that once, going to visit a housebound patient she suddenly became conscious that, as she said, '...we are helping Christ to carry His cross. I didn't think, Christ in the person of the sick — no, simply Christ.'

Hanna understood and internalised at a profound level the mystery of the nature of suffering and what it might mean for the sick and disabled and their families and carers. She often wrote about this ontological problem and frequently spoke about it to her nurses and volunteers. She would encourage them saying, 'Let us imitate Christ, who with the greatest love would bend over the sick person.'

She often witnessed the apparently pointless suffering of others and encountered much pain herself so it is not suprising that she was always very sensitive when she spoke about pain. She would say, 'What the Christian response to pain should be and what it is in any particular instance, are two different stories. This is a very sensitive and difficult subject.' Like Christ in the gospels, she encountered many suffering people,and as a nurse she naturally strove to give her patients some relief from pain. She wrote: 'The most profound and deepest level of understanding of the nature of suffering is in fact difficult to share [widely] with others, given the almost complete disappearance of a sense of sacrifice, including, I dare to say, among young people in religious orders. Therefore this leads to much anger and protestation and the continuous painful questioning,'Why?' She adds in another letter, 'Our work, which has evolved out of a need to help those who are suffering, has a clearly apostolic aspect to it.'

Towards the end of her life, Hanna wrote of her younger friend from Warsaw, Teresa Strzembosz, who had died of cancer in 1970, 'Not everyone is given the grace to look Death in the eye. The *Ars Morendi*, that art of dying well, which was given to Teresa S. is a rare grace and we have to respect that'; adding a bit later, 'We will all die at some point, and speaking personally, Thank God.' When Hanna's cancer returned and she realised that her own days were numbered she said to her close friends, 'Now I can begin to prepare for that greatest adventure of all'.

As noted earlier, Hanna worked closely with the Bishop, later Archbishop of Kraków, Karol Wojtyła, now Pope St John Paul II. In 1960, during Lent, for the first time Hanna invited Bishop Wojtyła to accompany her on her visits to 35 chronically ill patients in their homes. From that time on, he made a point of regularly visiting the chronically sick of his diocese. He repeated his Lenten visits first with Hanna and then with Alina Rumun, until his election as Pope in 1978. Inspired by Hanna, he established an annual *Day for the Sick* (known locally as *Dni Chorych*) in the Kraków diocese, during which he celebrated Mass for the intentions of all the sick in his diocese and he preached a special homily to them.

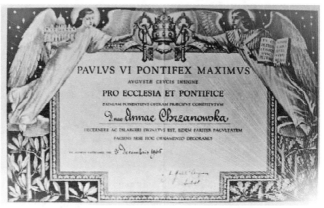

Papal Honour – Pro ecclesia et pontifice

It was also at the suggestion of Cardinal Wojtyła that in 1965, Pope Paul VI decorated Hanna with the *Pro Ecclesia et Pontifice* award in recognition of her work for the chronically ill and housebound in Kraków Diocese.

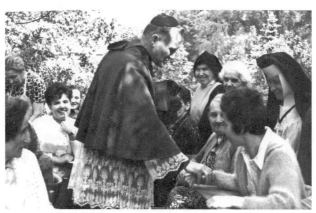

Cardinal Wojtyla in Trzebinia visiting the retreatants.

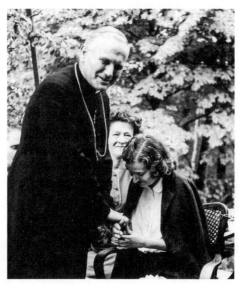

Cardinal Wojtyla in Trzebinia Retreat Centre with a participant

Concern for the sick and elderly was also typical of the future pope. Pope John Paul II began his ground breaking pontificate by arranging for his first trip outside the Vatican City to be a visit to his sick friend and senior colleague, Cardinal Deskur, at the Gemelli Clinic. Whenever Pope John Paul II made a pastoral visit, he made a point of meeting the chronically ill and disabled, and in 1992 he decreed that the feast of Our Lady of Lourdes, celebrated by the Roman Catholic Church on 11th February, be designated as a day when the universal Church prays for and with the ill, frail and disabled, and remembers those who care for them. He also visited the Marian shrine of Lourdes, which is known throughout the world for its message of compassionate care for the sick and handicapped, twice during his pontificate. He visited Lourdes for the last time in 2004, when he was a frail and ailing Bishop of Rome.

During his long pontificate he wrote and spoke about the nature of suffering; he also published an apostolic exhortation on suffering and the role of the sick in the life of the Church (*Salvifici Doloris*). He wrote in his autobiography that he owed much of his understanding of the suffering of the sick and his appreciation of their value to Hanna's work, life, and spirituality. When informed that the cause for her canonisation had been opened in Kraków, he responded with enthusiasm, saying that it was a good idea, which needed to be fostered.

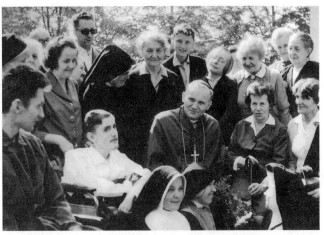

Volunteers, retreatants and Cardinal Karol Wojtyla.
Hanna is standing behind the Cardinal.

Meanwhile, one of Hanna's deliberate objectives was to draw both clergy and religious into her lay-led work. Although excited about her status as a member of the laity, she also wanted the clergy to take notice of the abandoned sick, those hidden away in the attics and basements of their parishes; she also wished that the sick might appreciate that the Church was concerned for their welfare. Cardinal Franciszek Macharski of Kraków 1927-2016 (who became archbishop of Kraków after the election of Karol Wojtyła to the See of Rome), observed Hanna's desire to educate clergy about the needs and spirituality of the sick. He said that Hanna would often remonstrate with him when he taught in Kraków seminary. Hanna said that he would only understand the mystery of suffering and the care of the sick when he spent time in hospital as a patient. He went on to become one of the most compassionate bishops of Kraków and was a firm supporter of Hanna. Several years later, the Cardinal Archbishop opened the cause for her canonisation.

As noted, Teresa Strzembosz was a Catholic social worker from Warsaw who had opened one of the first mother-and-child homes in Poland for single women. She was the instigator of the 1956 nurses' annual pilgrimage to Częstochowa, and she closely followed the developments of Parish Nursing in Kraków. Teresa wanted to establish similar parish-based care for the housebound in Warsaw.

In the autumn of 1960, Hanna sent Alina to Warsaw to work with Teresa and to show her how this could be done. It was no easier for Teresa to implement Parish Nursing in Warsaw than it had been for Hanna in Kraków, but due to Teresa's many contacts among nursing sisters in Warsaw, she managed to involve them in the project from the very beginning, especially the Daughters of Charity, who ran an inter-congregational nursing school in Warsaw. This was the only approved school of nursing that religious sisters in Poland were allowed to attend at that time; they were forbidden to attend government-run nursing schools. Meanwhile, Teresa, frustrated by some of the more reluctant priests and religious superiors, asked the Primate of Poland, now Venerable Servant of God Cardinal Stefan Wyszyński (1901–1981), to intervene and support the work. The cardinal immediately wrote to all the superiors and parish priests of the Diocese of Warsaw, urging them to stop hindering her work and to support Teresa's efforts to introduce Parish Nursing in Warsaw.

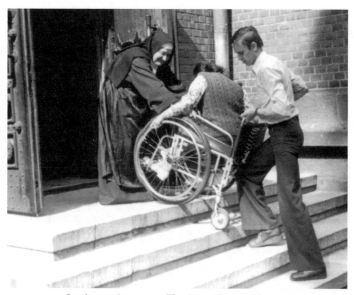

Student volunteer in Trzebinia Retreat Centre.

It was only a matter of time before Hanna started to organise retreats not only for her volunteers, but also for her patients, many of whom had not left their homes in years, if not decades. The first retreat Hanna organised for her housebound and wheelchair dependent patients was in 1964 in Trzebinia Retreat Centre, run by the Salvatorian Fathers. But for this work she needed additional help from young people. Professors and lecturers also came forward to help. Apart from medical help, professors, faculty members and various academics would also assist the project by making their telephones and cars available to Hanna. Many medical and university professors, who normally would not have participated in a church-related activity, happily agreed to help Hanna, transporting housebound patients to Trzebinia Retreat Centre in their cars. Some of them undertook this commitment for many years.

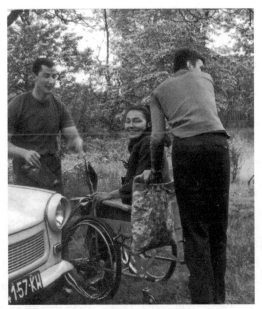

Students helping out in Trzebinia Retreat Centre.

Meanwhile, some students became involved for life, and would visit shut-ins and disabled patients for years afterwards, their lives permanently intertwined, often inter-generationally, with those of their new housebound friends... Students would read to the shut-ins, went to the cinema with young wheel-chair bound adolescents and even helped housebound handicapped youngsters get to school. One student noted, 'And it all started at St Anne's' — the chaplaincy church located in the university quarter, where Hanna had delivered an impassioned plea for help (essentially 'manpower') after a student Mass one Sunday. At the start of the project there were only a handful of students helping out in Trzebinia, but by the end there were hundreds. Word went round among the students that "Trzebiniacy" (those who went to Trzebinia), didn't fail their exams. This was enough encouragement for most students to want to lend a hand.

One woman started to cry as students carried her from her flat to be taken to Trzebinia Retreat Centre, where Hanna was organising these retreats. When asked why she was upset she answered, "I'm not upset. These are tears of joy because it's been years since I felt rain fall on my face!" Hanna was convinced of the need to take care of her patients in a variety of ways. She enabled them to attend retreats, Days of Prayer and, importantly, to have holidays. Today we would talk about the need for respite care. In the late 1950's and 1960's, the idea of integrating handicapped and chronically sick people into the mainstream of social and religious life in a diocese came close to an unachievable dream. Yet such dreams reflected the heartfelt desires of her patients, and Hanna knew this.

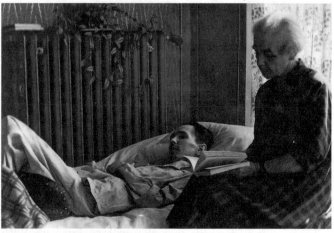

A volunteer reading to a housebound patient.

Writing about how to truly serve the chronically ill, she makes the point that we should not only give of ourselves in order to help them, but also be prepared to organise help from the outside, '...because the chronically ill housebound patient by the very nature of things has a limited range of experiences... The same four walls, the same ceiling, and so on.' This necessitates the organisation of additional help from a wider circle of people; it is reminiscent of the thoughtful care given by the Good Samaritan, '...Then he put the man on his own donkey, brought him to an inn and took care of him. The next day he took out two denarii and gave them to the innkeeper. 'Look after him,' he said, 'and when I return, I will reimburse you for any extra expense you may have.' (Lk 10:25-37)

Hanna's patients wanted to deepen their spiritual lives; but they also needed holidays, to experience a concert, or a day in the park. With her uncanny ability to listen and to elicit information from people, Hanna understood what they were asking for and searched for ways to respond to their needs. Today, such approaches to the care of the housebound and chronically sick are considered the norm for good pastoral outreach programmes and community projects for the sick and elderly. In Communist Poland fifty years ago, this was most unusual, and Hanna was far ahead of her time.

In 1971 Cardinal Karol Wojtyła nominated Hanna as coordinator and director of services for the handicapped and chronically ill for the Charities Commission of Kraków archdiocese. That same year, the Cardinal formally approved the regulations that were to govern the activities of parish nurses as members of a Church organisation as we have seen, which had been drawn up by Hanna, Teresa Strzembosz and her co-workers in 1966 and had been provisionally accepted.

Before the war in 1938, Hanna wrote an article for the Polish nursing journal about Fr Piotr Skarga, SJ, a 17th-century Polish Jesuit. Hanna greatly admired the saintly Jesuit and he was to have a profound influence on Hanna's nursing spirituality. Although a significant figure in Polish history and well known within the church in Kraków, only recently has his cause for canonisation been opened. He was a notable court preacher who also established Confraternities and Brotherhoods of Mercy in Kraków and Lwów, and other towns in southern Poland, to help distribute aid and care for the poor, sick, and abandoned. She commented in her article ' ...It is something especially precious and instructive to look back over three hundred years and discover in the magnificent work of Skarga many forms and methods of work which we would consider novel today. We find there not only exceptional organisation, excellent timetabling of work, with meticulous rationale, but above all, that without which any social work, even if it was consructed in the best way, would still bear no fruit — and that is a heart incandescent with love, which elevates the care of the poor to the heighest of Christian principles...' Hanna could have been writing that about her own approach to the care of the marginalised and abandoned in Kraków, three centuries after these recommendations by Piotr Skarga.

In a talk delivered in Warsaw, shortly before her death, Hanna outlined the three main aims of Parish Nursing: First, active demonstration of love for the sick; Second, penetration into human society — as a form of a loving initiative — a way of giving witness to Christ; and finally motivating and inspiring people of goodwill to engage with the sick. These three approaches reflect the activities of Christ on earth. First of all, Christ embodied goodness; he was full of mercy. Secondly, he went where noone else chose to go, so he touched those with leprosy, sat down to eat with sinners, and dared to talk with non-believers; and finally, he organised a community of believers. He taught his apostles and disciples, thus gathering around himself people willing to follow him — people who were prepared to continue his work. That is how Hanna tried to live and that was also her understanding of her role in Parish Nursing. Her Christ-centred, active Benedictine spirituality was based upon this gospel directive. She consciously lived out the recommendations on the role of the laity made by the Council fathers.

Hanna's idea of reaching out to the chronically ill and sick housebound was seen as an inspired response to an obvious nursing and social need. Hanna calculated that by 1970 the Parish Nursing project had looked after approximately 2,625 patients. This number included chronically ill individuals who were looked after by Hanna and her nurses for over twenty years. In 1973, she estimated that the Parish Nursing project was concerned with the healthcare and holistic needs of over 600 patients. It is amazing that all this care could have been coordinated and delivered before the era of cheap paper, pens, cardboard and medical supplies (all difficult to acquire in Socialist Poland), not to mention today's ubiquitous use of mobile phones, computers, easy access to cars or even landline telephones. Her work took place during some of the darkest days of Cold War Communism.

In 2004, in Lourdes, Pope St John Paul II said of the Blessed Virgin Mary, in his address to the pilgrims gathered there, 'Hers is *a practical love*, one which is not limited to words of understanding but is deeply and personally involved in giving help. The Blessed Virgin does not merely give her cousin something of herself; *she gives her whole self*, asking nothing in return. Mary understood perfectly that the gift she received from God is more than *a privilege*; it is a *duty* which obliges her to serve others with the selflessness proper to love.' This could also apply to Hanna, a woman for whom this Gospel story formed the foundation of her nursing work and who was so inspired by this Gospel narrative that it came to shape her life.

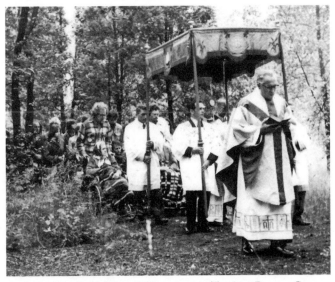

Procession with the Blessed Sacrament in Trzebini Retreat Centre. Note the disabled patients in the wheelchairs. The participants used to say that the highlight of the retreat was this procession and the blessing of the sick with the Blessed Sacrament – like in Lourdes.

CHAPTER 13

Colours of Fire: The Final Years 1966-1973

Blessed are the merciful for they shall have mercy shown them.
— Matthew 5:7

Hanna never enjoyed robust health. From early childhood, she spent weeks at a time in sanatoria and convalescent homes. As she grew older, allergies and intense sensitivity to drugs caused her considerable hardship. Knowledge about such sensitivity was minimal at that time, and antidotes to hyper-allergenic reactions were scarce.

Perhaps if Hanna had been less tired and had not pushed herself so hard, her body would not have reacted as violently as it did to noxious stimuli and chemical assaults. In the event, even a short visit to a friend or to a patient in hospital could cause her several days of acute distress. The very smell of hospital disinfectant caused her to have an acute allergic reaction. Nonetheless, she continued to visit sick relatives, patients and friends in hospital… life had to go on as normally as possible.

In 1966, as Catholic Poland was celebrating one thousand years of Christianity, Hanna realised she had serious health problems. Upon investigation she was diagnosed with an advanced gynaecological cancer. Aware of the gravity of the diagnosis, and in the absence of significant treatment other than surgery, she prepared herself for death. She was not afraid of death and wrote in a letter to a friend, '… What joy to be transported to that other world — sheer poetry.' She disposed of many of her possessions, wrote a will and, most interestingly, wrote a letter to her friend, Bishop Karol Wojtyła, stipulating that it was to be read after her death. But she recovered, and lived to spend her last eight years preparing, as she liked to say, for the 'greatest adventure of all.' Living on borrowed time, Hanna threw herself even more intensely into activities to do with Parish Nursing. This time, however, not only did she have *personal* knowledge of suffering but also a heightened awareness of the impending finality of her own life. This awareness coloured all her subsequent actions. In 1972, the cancer returned. Increasingly, she had to give up personal involvement in the direct care of others and delegated much of her work to her helpers, focusing more on nursing administration and writing.

As late as February 1973, two months before her death, she delivered a paper on Parish Nursing to the annual conference of the Polish Bishops' Commission on Church Charities in Warsaw. This report was an evaluation and summary of her work which perfectly reflected her mature nursing spirituality. But a year or so previously, she had written in a notebook, during a retreat for the sick in Trzebinia, the following prayer: 'Allow me to live here only for the sick, for You... And may I be, Oh Mother, under your care, safe under your cloak. Intercede for me, truly unfortunate with my uncontrolled nerves'. She added: '...I will not grumble any more about my lack of strength, and decreasing powers. After all, they are not disappearing into some unknown void. So let every greying hair be joyfully accepted, as an announcement of my journey towards you; as every step of my aching legs brings me ever closer to you, Father'.

Hanna, the committed Benedictine oblate and serious Christian was well aware of her imperfections and shortcommings and constantly working on her faults — as curbing her tongue, restraining her impatience, and concealing her disappointment when people let her down or things did not work out. As Dom Leon Knabit OSB observed at the 1993 conference in honour of Hanna, most things did in fact work out for Hanna, and with her charismatic personality most people were only too happy to help her, but she also experienced disappointment, and was sometimes let down, as she conveys in her prayer quoted above. This prayer may also indicate that she knew — before she told anyone else — that she was getting weaker and that her time on earth was limited.

As a competent nurse, she was well aware of her impending death. She wrote a more detailed version of her 1966 letter and final testament and had them sent to Cardinal Wojtyła; she also made detailed provision for disposing her goods, giving most of her possessions to friends and patients, not forgetting her family. Hanna gave her favourite book on mountain flora to her close friend and fellow Benedictine oblate, Wacława Bogdal, who also received her Oblate's scapular. She gave to one of her early patients Janina Hertz (who later became an author), a copy of her old treasured bible and a comfortable armchair in which to sit and read it. Mindful of the needs of her friends, Hanna left a damask tablecloth to her former student Irena Iżycka and asked her to take responsibility for the historical section of the Kraków branch of the Polish Nurses Association. She gave her co-worker and close oblate friend Alina Rumun a beautiful bone china tea cup... and so the list goes on. Those things which Hanna had inherited from her well-to-do relatives she arranged to pass on to her friends, knowing that in Communist Poland of the 1970s, these items were unavailable, even if one had the money to buy them. To this day, Hanna's various gifts are enjoyed and used, and some are now in museums.

Hanna's material preparations for death were meticulous and thoughtful. She even placed in her wardrobe the dress and shoes she wished to wear for her burial. Everything else she gave away. She wanted her death to be as stress-free as possible for her friends and relatives. But Hanna's chief legacy to her co-workers was a nursing spirituality which still resonates among nurses and healthcare workers. As she once said, 'Let us not just think about fighting evil. It may well be that evil absorbs us more — and not just as a literary subject. We must talk about it, of course, even shout about it. But can't we also shout about goodness? About that goodness, which is born out of misery, and is being created anew by Love, day after day. Surely what I have observed [during my lifetime] are not just phantom shades. I see it all so clearly now – in the vivid colours of fire!'

In early March 1973, Hanna went to rest in the Tatra Mountains with Alina Rumun and some friends, as she usually did each spring; but by now her health was fading.

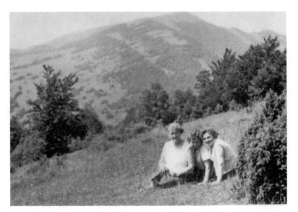

Hanna in the Polish Tatra Mountains.

On her return to Kraków she barely had the strength to climb the stairs to her second-floor apartment and once she reached her flat, she was never to leave it. During the last few weeks of Hanna's life, as pain increasingly caused her discomfort, friends started to visit her more frequently in order to say their goodbyes. She received the Sacrament of the Sick from Fr Franciszek Macharski, who had been appointed by Cardinal Karol Wojtyła as chaplain to healthcare workers in the Kraków region. She made her final Confession and received the Holy Eucharist. As we have seen, Fr Franciszek was also a close friend of Hanna's and a staunch supporter of her work. He had often led the retreats and Days of Prayer which Hanna organised. After her death, and following the election of Karol Wojtyła to the See of Rome, he was nominated Cardinal Archbishop of Kraków.

At this time Hanna found solace from having her friends read to her from the Scriptures, and unsurprisingly her favourite passage was the opening verses of St John's Gospel – '*In the beginning was the Word, and the Word was with God, and the Word was God.*' She repeatedly listened to these words and meditated on them. Soon however, visits even by close friends began to tire her and according to Alina Rumun, the only person whose visits she still looked forward to were those of Cardinal Wojtyła, who visited several times.

Although according to Alina, Hanna lost some of her character-istic humour and joy, for she was in considerable pain, she still retained her typical directness. One evening as two of her parish nurses started to argue, at the foot of her bed, about which pads and gauzes to use, Hanna, who until that point lay quietly in the bed with her eyes closed, opened her eyes and looking straight at them said in the authoritative voice of a nursing lecturer — 'Here I am dying, while you two are squabbling about gauzes! Stop.'

Meanwhile, spring was approaching, and Cardinal Wojtyła was informed of Hanna's rapidly deteriorating health. He too, paid Hanna one last visit to bless and console his friend. Wacława Bogdal relates that she was caring for Hanna at the time, and the Cardinal's visit caused a stir in the apartment. The Cardinal asked if he could be left alone with Hanna, but every so often he would come rushing out of her room, looking for Wacława saying '…Hanna wants something.' Finally, at the end of the visit the Cardinal asked Wacława, if it would be possible for both of them to move Hanna up in the bed and make her more comfortable.

Although the Cardinal had a much younger priest waiting for him outside (probably his escort driver), he wanted to help Hanna himself. He tucked up his sleeves and, following Wacława's directions, helped to re-position Hanna. This was his last act of kindness towards her. It was the same act of good nursing that he had witnessed Hanna perform so many times for her patients, and it illustrates how normal and unceremonious were the relationships that Hanna fostered among her friends, both nurses and clergy.

Just before daybreak on 29 April 1973, the day on which the Roman Catholic Church celebrates the feast of Saint Catherine of Siena (c1347–1380), Hanna died in her flat on Łobzowska Street. Catherine of Siena, the quintessentially active secular Dominican woman, politically aware, yet quietly contemplative, was an appropriate saint to accompany Hanna on her journey to heaven. Although Hanna was a Benedictine oblate and Catherine was a Dominican tertiary, this wise medieval woman inspired and engaged men and women, clergy and laity, to care for others in a way similar to Hanna.

Additionally, that year, 29 April was the first Sunday after Easter, known today as Mercy Sunday. This feast which concludes the Easter octave was instituted for the universal Church by Pope St John Paul II in April 2000, a feast which was advocated by another mystic from Kraków — St Faustyna Kowalska. Hanna, who strove to be merciful to so many people in so many different ways during her eventful and busy life, was now to receive God's infinite mercy and love — for eternity.

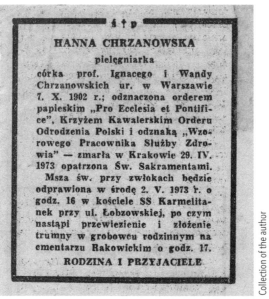

Obituary for Hanna Chrzanowska in local Kraków newspaper, sent in by her family and friends. After her name is written: Pielęgniarka – Nurse.

Hanna found the strength for her nursing work in attendance at daily Mass and in quiet daily prayer, often in the Carmelite monastery across the road from her apartment. The nuns knew her well, and supported her work with their prayers; sometimes they even prepared meals for her, as Hanna was often too busy to cook for herself. It is no suprise then, that it was decided to celebrate the requiem Mass for Hanna in the nuns' chapel. The funeral was scheduled for the 2nd May. The day was a beautiful, warm spring day; which heralded the joys of summer. For Hanna it heralded a whole new life. The Cardinal Archbishop of Kraków, Karol Wojtyła, insisted on presiding at the concelebrated Eucharist, despite the fact that in order to do so he missed a plenary session of the Polish Episcopal Congress, meeting in Wrocław. He also accompanied her coffin to the Rakowicki Cemetery.

At the graveside, he read aloud extracts from the letter which he had received from Hanna in 1966, when she was first diagnosed with cancer. In it Hanna asked the Cardinal to tell her colleagues and friends to continue the work which she had started, to trust in their own abilities and never to forget the needs of the housebound and chronically ill. The Cardinal added: 'We thank the merciful God for your life, and let your reward be the Lord Himself; let the radiance of your service linger among us and be a constant example, teaching us how to serve Christ in our neighbours.'

It is a testimony to Hanna's uniqueness that the funeral Mass took place within the Carmelite monastery chapel, instead of her local parish church, or the cemetery chapel, which would have been the normal practice. Also, in a spontaneous break with tradition at the end of the service at the cemetery, the Cardinal intoned the *Magnificat*, the song of joy and thanksgiving sung by Mary upon greeting her cousin Elizabeth during the Visitation. This gesture was yet another example of one of those 'quiet miracles' that marked Hanna's life. As we have seen, she had a great fondness for the Gospel story of young Mary *hurrying* to visit her older cousin Elizabeth, who — according to the news of the angel — was now with child. Hanna liked to say to her colleagues and friends, 'I need to go in haste — as Mary did — to answer the needs of my patients. We need to go in haste and we must not linger…'

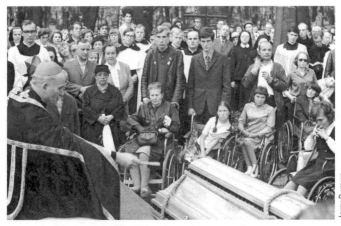

Jerzy Rumun

Cardinal Wojtyla at the graveside.

So, when the time came to bid Hanna farewell from this world, the Cardinal intoned the Marian hymn — the *Magnificat*. Hanna was now at rest, and together with those at the cemetery she too affirmed with the Mother of Christ that 'The Almighty works marvels for me. Holy his name! His mercy is from age to age, on those who fear him.' (Lk 1:48-50)

CHAPTER 14

A Reflection of the Goodness of God:
A Nursing Spirituality and Legacy

'Don't call me a saint. I don't want to be dismissed so easily.'
— Dorothy Day

Hanna Chrzanowska, who was well known in Poland during her lifetime, became a legend after her death. Several homes for the disabled and frail elderly have taken Hanna as their patron and a newly-established children's hospice in Kraków is named after her. At present, six schools for allied health professionals have chosen Hanna as their patron and are named after her. The Kraków Nursing School preserves much archival material and mementoes from the time of her work there, ranging from letters, documents, and notes to manuscripts, furniture, and even tea-cups. Many of these are now displayed in a university departmental museum. Needless to say, the present Kraków School of Nursing, which is a separate department of the Jagiellonian University, is enormously proud of its connection with Hanna.

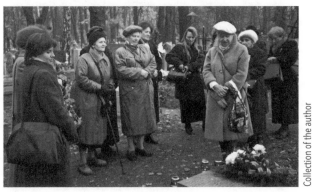

Collection of the author

Kraków nurses, among them many of Hanna's past students'
praying at her graveside.

She was not forgotten by her co-workers and nursing friends and memorial Masses were often said for her. A few years after Hanna died, there was a memorial Mass on the anniversary of her death. During the reception afterwards in the cloisters of the Kraków Franciscan church, Zofia Szlendak-Cholewińska, a community nursing colleague of Hanna's from the Kraków School of Nursing pointed out to her friends that much was being said about the specialness of Hanna and about her evident holiness, but little was being done about it.

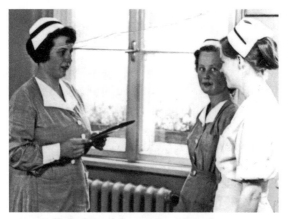

Zofia Szlendak at work with students.

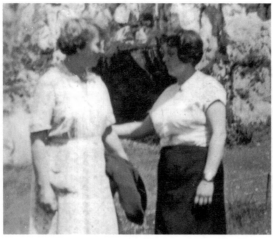

Zofia Szlendak with Hanna in Tyniec

Zofia recalled that a couple of years after Hanna's death, Dom Piotr Rostworowski from Tyniec Abbey, who had known both Hanna and Zofia quite well, as he had been their spiritual director for a while, had come to visit her and they talked long into the evening about Hanna's work and her holiness. But Zofia had formerly been a member of a secular institute, which she later left. She moved away from the Church and although most of her former friends severed their relationships with her, Dom Piotr still kept in contact with her. Dom Piotr said to Zofia at the time that if Hanna was ever to be beatified, then the initiative would need to come from the nurses themselves. Given Zofia's strained relationship with the Church, this seemed to her such a remote possibility, that she was amused, and dismissed the advice as fanciful. She did not imagine that she would end up playing a crucial part in the beatification of Hanna.

A few more years went by and in May 1993, the Executive Council of the Catholic Nurses and Midwives Association of Poland and the Kraków Regional Division of the Polish Nurses' Association jointly organised a conference in honour of Hanna. This was to commemorate the twentieth anniversary of her death and to acquaint a new generation of nurses with the story of her life. It was also an opportune moment to express an appreciation of Hanna by those who still remembered her: nurses, patients, volunteers and friends alike.

By this time Zofia had completely moved away from the Faith; her church attendance lapsed as she aggressively chose a different path. But while Zofia had pointed out the inactivity of her colleagues in regards to promoting Hanna's canonisation cause, her own unwitting role in facilitating Hanna's beatification was just beginning. It was her remarks in the Franciscan cloisters, to her nursing friends, several years previously, which eventually prompted the Kraków branch of the Catholic Association of Nurses to approach Cardinal Macharski about the canonisation of Hanna.

The nurses organising the conference remembered Zofia's question from a few years' earlier, and people present at the gathering also agreed that something should be done about Hanna's cause, so it was decided that they would approach Cardinal Franciszek Macharski, Archbishop of Kraków about their resolution to see their 'special' colleague included among the saints of the church. They knew she was a holy woman but they wanted the rest of the world to know that also and to learn from Hanna's way of life. Hanna was an inspiration and a role model for the nurses and they wanted this to be formally recognised. The Cardinal who knew Hanna well, agreed with them.

In May 1998, another major conference was held to commemorate the 25th anniversary of Hanna's death and at that meeting, more reports and stories were heard about the significance of Hanna's life. The Catholic Nurses' Association (Kraków Branch) was formally entrusted with helping to collect and organise material concerning Hanna for the Archdiocese of Kraków, which had opened the cause for her canonisation on 3 November 1998, at the specific request of the nurses who knew Hanna so well and who had worked with her.

A couple of years later, Zofia (now completely estranged from the Catholic faith), decided to go to the Rakowicki cemetery in order to visit the grave of her husband and of 'Auntie' (as the Kraków nurses affectionately referred to Hanna). She suddenly felt an urge to pray but realised that she had forgotten the words of the prayer Our Father. As Zofia later told the promoters of Hanna's canonisation, this terrified her, that she, who once recited the prayer several times a day, had forgotten the words which once meant so much to her. She started to violently cry and shouted over Hanna's grave, 'Hanna save me'.

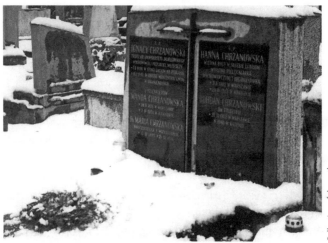

Collection of the author

Hanna's original grave in Rakowicki Cemetery, Kraków

During the previous years, Zofia had strange blackouts and pseudo-epileptic seizures. There were periods when she was constantly falling over and losing her balance, resulting in several broken limbs. She even once fell in front of a tram. Finally, after exhaustive tests she was diagnosed with a massive cerebral aneurism for which there was no medicine or surgery possible.

One day in March 2001, on an impulse, a close friend of Zofia's from the Kraków School of Nursing and an active member of the Catholic Nurses' Association, Anna Putko, one of the few nurses who had not severed ties with Zofia, telephoned her to find out how she was. Zofia replied, 'I'm not feeling too good but don't bother to come to me tonight, for the night is sacred. Come and visit me tomorrow.' Anna considered this an odd thing for Zofia to say, since Zofia was no longer a practising Catholic and did not normally use such pious or poetic language. That night the aneurism burst and Zofia was rushed to hospital with a slim chance of survival, or if she did survive the night, with catastrophic residual damage. Zofia remained in a coma for six weeks.

During the time that Zofia was in hospital, the Association of Catholic nurses were praying for her recovery and her spiritual healing through Hanna's intercession. They held a novena of prayers for Zofia's intention with exposition of the Blessed Sacrament, in the nurses' church of St Nicholas. During the novena, Anna Putko once again felt an urgent need to leave the church and visit Zofia in the hospital to see how she was. Upon arrival, she was amazed to see that Zofia had fully recovered consciousness and was talking clearly and asking for a priest! Zofia later recounted how she saw Hanna appear to her just as she was losing consciousness and that Hanna had reassured her that all would be well.

Anna Putko said that it was incredible to watch Zofia recover from the burst aneurism, in an exceptionally short time. Remarkably, there was no evidence of damage to Zofia's brain tissue, and no evidence of the cerebral trauma which Zofia had experienced over the previous several years. On the new brain scans, only a tiny scar showed up — as if to tease the puzzled neurologists. Zofia regained full use of all her limbs and faculties.

In fact she functioned better after the miraculous cure, than before the massive cerebral aneurism. The doctors had no explanation for the sudden and permanent healing of Zofia. However a greater cure was the healing of Zofia's soul. According to Anna, Zofia cried in pain and in joy when she was taken down to the hospital chapel, because she had been brought back into the fold of the Good Shepherd. She cried throughout the entire Mass, and received Holy Communion for the first time, in several decades.

In 2015, the Congregation for the Cause of Saints in Rome formally decreed that Hanna had practised the theological virtues of Faith, Hope and Charity to a heroic degree, and could be officially referred to as a Venerable Servant of God. On 6 April 2016 the mortal remains of Hanna were removed from the Rakowicki cemetery, identified, and laid in a new coffin in the crypt of St Nicholas' Church on Kopernika Street, in the heart of the Kraków hospital district, an area well known to Hanna throughout her working life.

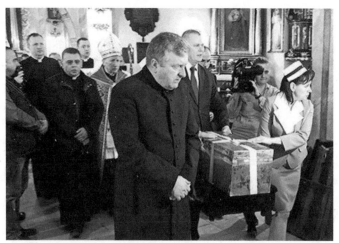

Translation of the relics of Venerable Servant of God Hanna
Chrzanowska from the Rakowicki Cemetery to the church of St Nicholas.

The church of St Nicholas has been designated for several years now as the official nurses' church in Kraków and it currently serves as the headquarters of the Kraków branch of the Catholic Nurses and Midwives Association. It is from this church that the pastoral work with the nurses of Kraków is conducted.

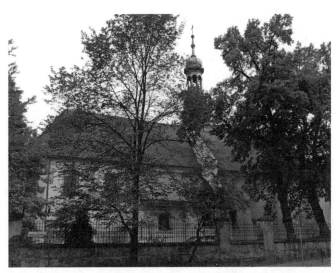

Church of St Nicholas, Kraków

The church was first mentioned in an official papal document written by Pope Gregory IX to the Benedictine monks of Tyniec Abbey in 1229, and is described there as a chapel located outside the walls of the medieval town. It would appear to have been one of the chapels belonging to the monastic community. By 1327, it had already become a parish church. In 1456, the church and its lands were given by the abbey to the Jagiellonian University. In one of those unexplainable coincidences of divine intervention, this medieval church with connections both to the Benedictine abbey of Tyniec and the Jagiellonian University, is now to become the final resting place of Hanna, a Benedictine oblate of Tyniec Abbey, a place closely connected through her own studies and work, and of course her father, with the ancient university. The church is also notable because on the 13th April 1884, Emila Kaczorowska was baptised there. She was to become the future mother of Pope St John Paul II.

On the 7th July 2017, the cardinals in Rome accepted the cure of Zofia Szlendak-Cholewińska, attributed to the intercession of Hanna, as miraculous, and Pope Francis confirmed that she could be beatified, in her home town of Kraków. Hanna, who in her memoirs commented about herself that, '…she was no saint', was officially declared by Cardinal Angelo Amato of the Congregation for the Causes of Saints and in the presence of Polish cardinals and bishops and the Kraków Archdiocese, to be a *Blessed* of the Roman Church on the 28th April 2018; it was almost 45 years to the day, from the date of her birth to heaven.

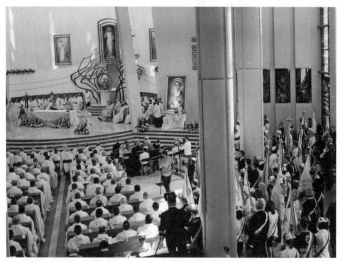

Beatification ceremony of Bl. Hanna Chrzanowska

Marie Romagnano

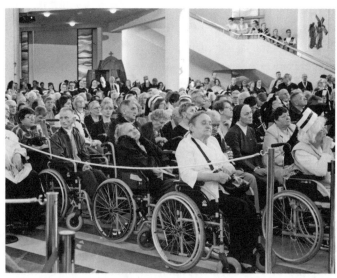

Special guests at the ceremony

Marie Romagnano

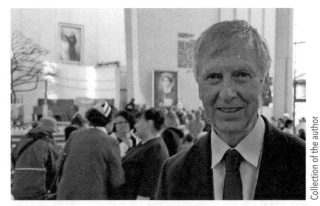

Collection of the author

Godson and nephew of Blessed Hanna, Mr Stanisław Karol Szlenkier
after the Beatification Ceremony 28th April 2018

Present at the ceremony were also Polish nursing dignitaries
from Warsaw and nurses from schools and establishments around
Poland named after Hanna, and who consider Hanna to be their
patron; also regular practising nurses from Kraków, especially from
the Kraków branch of the Catholic Nurses Association. In addition,
attending the ceremony was Miss Geraldine McSweeney — president
of CICIAMS — representing Catholic nurses from around the world;
and Mrs Marie Romagnano representing nurses and Healthcare Professionals for Divine Mercy, from the USA. Together with the author
of this book they went in procession carrying their lit nursing oil-
lamps, following immediately behind the Vice-postulator of Hanna's
canonisation cause, Mme Helena Matoga, who carried a grand golden
reliquary containing a relic of Blessed Hanna.

Blessed Hanna's mortal remains are now contained in an alabaster sarcophagus bought and designed by the nurses of Poland, and
located in the chapel of St Anne in St Nicholas' Church. The nurses'
church of St Nicholas now houses the shrine containing the mortal
remains of a saintly woman, who was outstanding for her works of
mercy and goodness. The presence of her relics in the church is a gift to
nurses around the world, who can pray at Blessed Hanna's tomb and
call that church their home. On the 28th of every month formal prayers
are said and the Holy Mass is celebrated by her shrine, for the many
intentions listed in the book of requests. Blessed Hanna's feast is to be
celebrated on the 28th April.

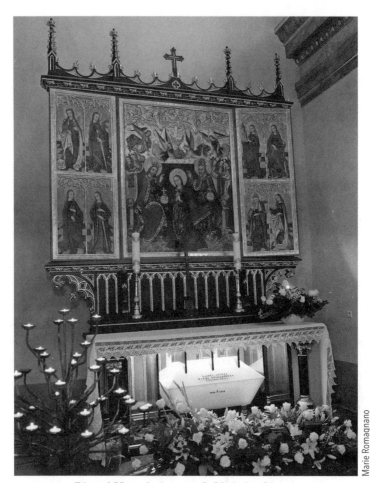

Blessed Hanna's shrine in St Nicholas Church

Hanna is now one step closer to being declared a saint of the universal church — someone who from heaven will continue to help and inspire nurses, oblates, social workers, and many others, to lead a deeper and more Christ-centred life. Just as during her lifetime, when Hanna looked after the welfare of her nurses, so from heaven she responded to the cries of her nursing friend Zofia. Hanna now continues to point the way for nurses, oblates, and many others to follow Christ — reminding them to seek the welfare of others and to help each other in love, while not forgetting to support each other in prayer.

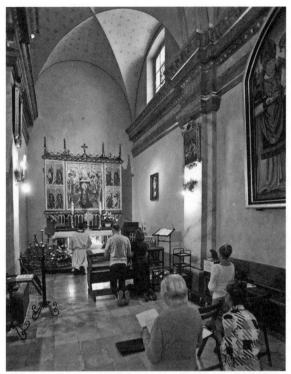

Praying at the shrine of Blessed Hanna in St Nicholas' Church.

Hanna was a woman who worked miracles of loving, active compassion in a Communist country which would have willingly imprisoned her for anti-socialist activities; and yet she worked openly as a practising Catholic nurse, bringing solace, joy and a degree of normality to hundreds of housebound invalids whom the world had forgotten about and had marginalised. She mobilised others to help her establish parish nursing without any of the modern conveniences which we now take for granted. During her life she profoundly influenced hundreds of people in Kraków and other parts of Poland, from Karol Wojtyła (now Pope St John Paul II) to countless patients, nurses and university student volunteers. As noted already, at least two young people who worked as volunteers with Hanna's Parish Nursing project (a nurse — Janina Wojnarowska and an engineer — Jerzy Ciesielski), are today considered as candidates for sainthood, while she had a lively friendship with several more individuals who are now being considered for canonisation, such as Maria Epstein, (Sister Magdalena OP). This was a true communion of saints. It is hoped that once Hanna is canonised, she will influence and inspire, many more nurses, oblates, and ordinary folk not only in Poland, but also around the world, to follow the call of the Gospel as she did, and fall in love with Christ.

Her Christian vocation — her path to heaven — was lived out as a qualified registered nurse — no more, no less. Her unique spirituality was a *nursing* spirituality and her particular manifestation of holiness is seen in her abandonment of self in the service of the sick poor — that is, to Christ among us. Hanna was empowered and energised through her service to others. She found herself closest to God and entered most fully into the richness of being human as she restored dignity to those around her. For Hanna, it was predominantly people and a love of nature which provided the impetus and meditative force behind her experience of God, a sentiment beautifully captured in her poem *Cross on the Sand*. She reaffirms with all creation that, '...*be praised Lord in your rainbow, And amidst the scent of lupines, For the choirs of birds – like the seraphim, Echo your greatness.*'

In her nursing vocation Hanna discovered her truest self, and she consciously accepted her vocation as a gift from God. She understood that this was her specific road to the Lord, appreciating that her whole life was already given over to Him, that she belonged to Him, and that everything she did was done for love of Him. In a letter she wrote in 1971 to Cardinal Archbishop Wojtyła she said, "I am eternally grateful to God that he specifically chose me to do this [work]. That he surprised me — dazzled me. That here on earth he showed me his mercy, forgave me so many wrongs which I performed against him, for such a long time, in my complicated life. The fact that He threw me into this work with the sick is evidence enough of his pardon and grace. As I well know, God is a whirlwind of Love. And by telling me to serve in this format and no another, He dropped me into His whirlpool, His whirlwind, like a tiny leaf, a bit of dust only circling around the edges — but all the same, caught up in the motion, the unimaginable motion of Love."

Hanna considered nursing to be her vocation, not only in the secular professional sense, as a physician or artist might have a vocation to a particular type of work; she considered it to be a sacred calling. Indeed, Hanna regarded her nursing activities as a reflection and consequence of a particular nursing spirituality. She stated in a conference to a group of nurses that: '… the very fact of having chosen our profession, our very acceptance of this service, is simultaneously, as long as we are also Catholic, an acceptance of our vocation from God.' Hanna had no illusions about her call to be a nurse, even though, as she pointed out in her memoirs, there were some very human circumstances that pushed her into that discipline. Grace always builds on nature.

Hanna intuitively realised that just as the human person is holy, by virtue of the mystery of the Incarnation, so nursing work is sanctifying, both for the patient and the nurse. Indeed the very work environment was to be considered as a sacred place, fleas and all, because it is the arena where the patient, the nurse, and Christ meet. Hanna moved away from the compartmentalised model of the world which sees everything divided into neat spheres of the sacred or profane. Hanna demonstrated that all life is sacred and all nursing work which supports that life is to be considered sacred also. She demonstrated an empowering lay Benedictine spirituality which she lived out almost exclusively within the definitions of her highly visible professional nursing activities, while simultaneously leading a deeply hidden and profoundly personal prayer-life. Hanna never felt the need to be a religious sister; she considered her professional nursing activities as a sufficient vocation.

Hanna's spirituality and womanly wisdom were manifested through the many activities of her busy professional and personal life. Her spirituality was not something added onto her life as an optional extra; rather, it was an integral aspect of her Christian, feminine and nursing way of being. Indeed, her wise caring can only be adequately judged in relation to the totality of her life and the Christian values for which she stood.

In conclusion, Hanna's spirituality was a reflection of her Christian professional life, which she lived to the full in a mostly war-torn and weary Europe. She turned towards the ancient Benedictine tradition for prayerful inspiration and support which sustained and motivated her to continue in her gruelling professional and pastoral work, in a hostile Communist country, in the context of a mainly pre-conciliar Church. As Pope St John Paul II remarked, she started, '…a new "creativity" in charity work'. Such a vibrant and healthy spirituality must have required a considerable measure of wisdom and love to flourish; and, if nothing else, Hanna Chrzanowska was a wise woman and a compassionate nurse. She was a saint.

Works by Blessed Hanna

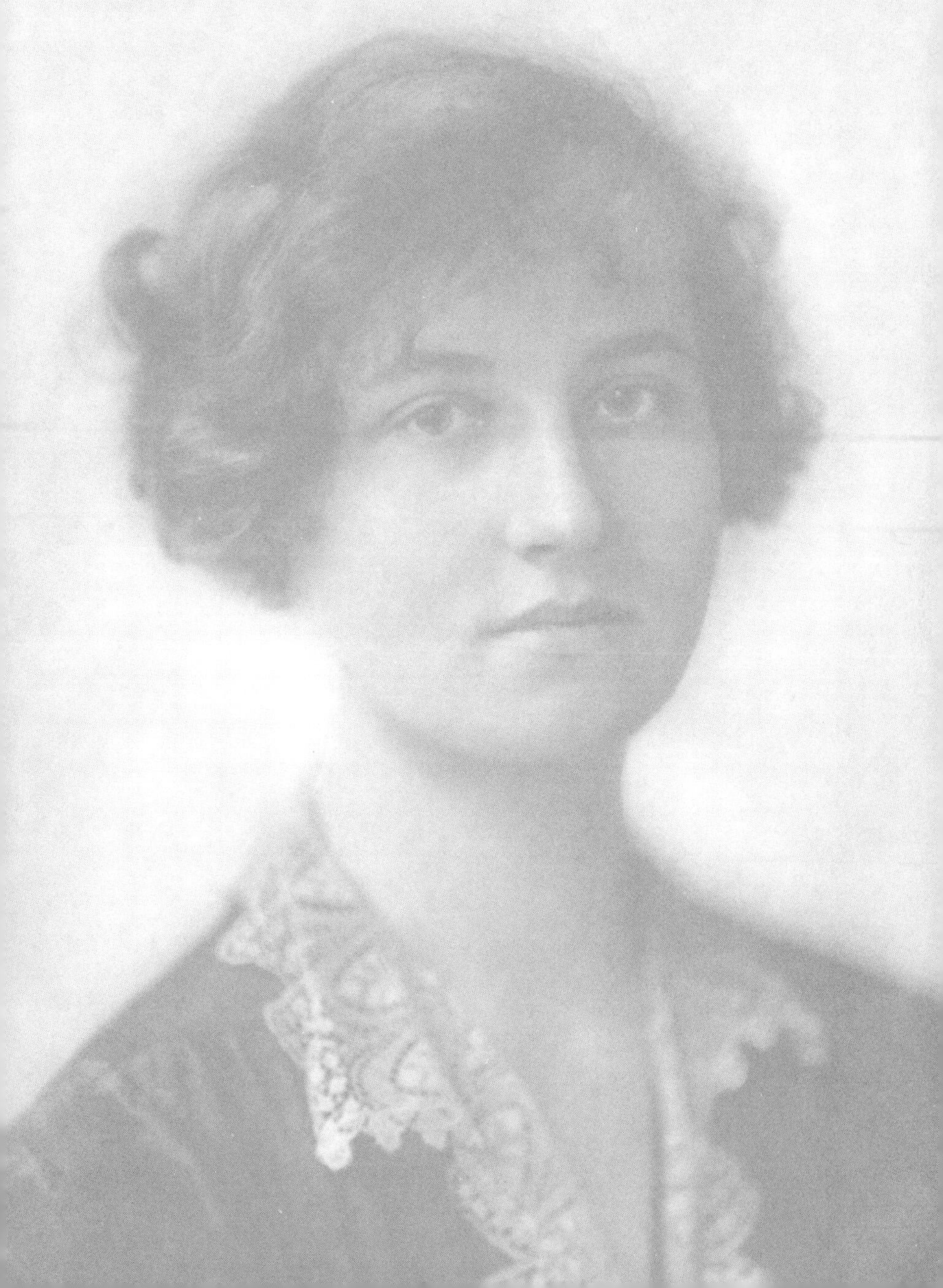

A Cross on the Sand

Bl. Hanna Chrzanowska

I do not know my Lord,
How much more time you have prepared for me.
Maybe I will not go down to the woods today –
The pine-woods.

Maybe the sound of the heaven-bound skylark
Will not reach me anymore?
Or maybe I will not finish this prayer – or see the sun again;
Because today's rains
May last an eternity for me?
Or perhaps you are preparing for me
many more long years, all in a long row;
So very long…

Till the hairs on my head will be smothered
In a blanket of whiteness, like the first snow.
Do not therefore spurn me
That I wish to bend Your Son's prayer
"Thy will be done "
Into a quiet plea:
That the hand of death may not alter
The sharpness of my vision,
And that I may still gaze with joy
On the vastness of your cosmic spaces.
That I will not cry out, bent double with human grief
When dying,
Because I shall never see again
The green freshness of the fields.

So be praised Lord in your rainbow
And amidst the scent of lupines,
For the choirs of birds – like the seraphim
Echo your greatness.

Translated from Polish by Gosia Brykczyńska

A Nurse's Examination of Conscience

Bl. Hanna Chrzanowska

Part I

1. I am a nurse. I'm a Catholic. Can I say with a clear conscience: "I am a Catholic nurse"?

2. My job is not only my profession but also my vocation. I will understand more fully this vocation if I enter into and make my own Christ's words, "I did not come to be served, but to serve".

3. I must fulfil my vocation to the best of my ability, mindful of any family responsibilities which I may also have; performing my nursing work in a spirit of service and love.

4. God has put talents in my hands and I must not waste them. Christ Himself through His activities among the sick shows me how to behave.

Part II

1. Every act of Christ's mercy was a manifestation of holiness. In spite of this Christ would still retire from people in order to pray. Do I follow His example? Do I delude myself thinking that my work is my 'prayer'? And yet I have time for so many other activities outside of work! Can I really not find some time just for God? Do I pray for strength? Do I thank God for my vocation?

2. Do I neglect Holy Mass on Sundays and feast days, convincing myself that I too tired?

3. Do I try to get to know my religion more deeply through reading, discussions, or attending religious conferences? If not — why? Because of arrogance or laziness? Maybe I do not want to hear the truth about myself?

4. Do I remember that God looks at me and sees everything? Am I only working to make an impression, to gain praise, or to dazzle those working with me?

5. The good which I achieve is only a reflection of the goodness of God. Have I boasted about my work? Do I overly admire myself?

6. Do I work on developing in myself the qualities of a good nurse and not become discouraged in this undertaking?

Part III

1. Do I appreciate the dignity of my profession and do I try to express it in words and deeds? Do I understand that going beyond my nursing duties and reaching for the physician's role can be a departure from the path of my calling?

2. As a Catholic nurse, do I feel co-responsibility for my profession? What am I doing to raise its status profile? Do I evade professional involvement in this area?

3. If I am married, and I have children, and yet work professionally, how do I combine both responsibilities? As a nurse, am I sufficiently committed that my personal concerns do not jeopardize those patients entrusted to my care, be they in the hospital or the clinic or in the community? Or — alternatively — do I neglect my family responsibilities in preference for my work? Perhaps I am taking on too much work, immersing myself in it unnecessarily? Am I cheerful and polite only at work, but then unwind at home in a foul irritable mood? Or maybe it's the other way round?

4. How do I fulfil my professional duties; am I punctual, conscientious in carrying out orders. Do I work according to the principles of the art of nursing in the hospital, clinic, and in the patient's home?

5. Maybe I work with modern equipment, among the most advanced achievements of medicine. Do I remember that these inventions and scientific achievements reflect the glory of God, the Creator of human thought? Do I try to continually improve myself professionally?

6. Am I truthful? Do I have the courage to admit my errors and

mistakes, or maybe not, concealing or falsifying facts to protect my actions or my convictions? Was I conscientious in my verbal and written reports, documentation, and statistics?

7. Do I respect common property? Have I destroyed it or misappropriated it? Have I returned everything I have borrowed?

8. What is my attitude towards my own welfare and the welfare of my colleagues? Do I have the courage to intervene with legitimate demands for improvement? Do I take part in strikes or have I encouraged others to participate? Have I received money or other remuneration dishonestly? This could have been in the form of 'compensation' or a bonus upon leaving a hospital, or for complaining about harsh conditions. Did I take money in advance "to better care for a hospital patient", or did I negotiate a fee with a family for compensation later, while on a salary; do I understand that this is simply a bribe? Do I suggest the use of medications which I want to promote, although they are not needed? Perhaps I ask too high a price for medicines which I received for sale? Maybe I demanded too high a fee for private practice, not taking into account the financial resources of the sick? Despite a low salary do I work without reproach?

9. How do I respond to the request to work extra hours — in the case of standing in for someone, or an epidemic, or the need for additional home visits, or staying on with a seriously ill patient?

10. Do I have anything to admit in regards to my behaviour towards staff and patients of the opposite sex? If everything is fine at work, what about in my private life? Do I understand that the Lord God does not divide morality into "private" and "work-related" spheres and that His commandments are immutable?

11. Do I look after for my own health? Do I exhaust myself unnecessarily, claiming recklessly that "Nothing will happen to me"? Is my life-style undermining my strength to work?

Part IV

1. What is my attitude towards a person who is ill? Do I make a conscious effort not to fall into apathy and routine?

2. Do I pray for the sick and all those entrusted to my care?

3. Do I shy away from essential nursing care of the sick, resorting to more advanced and 'effective' treatments, unnecessarily replacing doctors?

And yet our patients sense our love the most, when we wash them, feed them, make them more comfortable! Do I do everything within my power to provide the sick with just such care, either personally or by skillfully organizing my own tasks or the work of others? Maybe I excuse myself from these genuine nursing tasks convincing myself that I need to do something else, or by specifically searching out something else to do, for example, tidying up the first aid kit — one more time, or writing out medical histories for the benefit of doctors? Perhaps I go to watch interesting procedures at the cost of neglecting the sick?

In community nursing — maybe I convince myself that I do not have the time to make another home visit, but still manage to create for myself the task of unnecessarily tidying up nursing reports?

4. Do I treat the sick simply as numbers, as sickness "cases" forgetting about the unique personality of each one of them? Do I remember that the hundredth surgery for me, is the first one for the patient? That every newborn baby — from among many — which I am carrying out [of the nursery] to his or her mother, is her greatest love?

5. Do I nurse with increased gentleness unconscious patients, children and the elderly? Do I encompass with special care the distressed and anxious?

6. What is my attitude towards the dying? When there is no one present from their family with them do I do everything I can to substitute for them? Were there occasions when I sat idly in the nurses' station, leaving dying patients to themselves?

7. How do I approach the religious concerns of the sick? Do I care for them? Was I maybe too insistent, following some set ideology? Did I do everything in my power to enable a seriously ill patient to receive the Holy Sacraments (e.g. Reconciliation, Anointing of the Sick, Viaticum and an Apostolic Pardon)? Am I concerned about baptism for Christian infants threatened with death? What is my collaboration

with the hospital chaplain like? Do I facilitate the chaplain's work by providing, whenever possible, peace in the patients' room, providing explanations, and sharing insights?

8. What is my attitude towards the family of my patient? Do I try to understand them? Was I patient with them even when they seemed boring and intrusive to me? What if it was my own child who was sick, or my father?

9. What is my attitude towards those I visit at home? Do I carry out my visits conscientiously and with kindness? Do I get discouraged by my lack of success? When I come across a chronically sick patient during home visits, do I try and care for them?

10. Do I maintain professional confidentiality not only in regards to the diagnosis of the disease, but also concerning the worries and problems entrusted to me by patients and their families while visiting in their homes?

11. Do I try to make procedures as painless as possible for the patients? Do I expose the sick unnecessarily, not respecting their modesty or that of other adults and children who may be present?

12. Do I understand that my duties include caring for the psychological nature of the sick? Do I try to find time to talk to them, am I patient enough? Do I try to entertain an ill child? Do I try and create a peaceful and pleasant atmosphere for the sick?

13. Do I let them feel my fatigue and haste? Have I given my patients promises without being fully aware that I may be unable to keep them? Do I keep my promises?

14. Did I anticipate their wishes and show them genuine care and concern? Do I remember that Christ acted immediately among his sick people, without delay, going out to meet them — and that the Mother of God went about her tasks "in haste"?

15. Do I display less of a caring attitude towards those sick people, whom I do not have much sympathy for, than for those with whom I can empathize? Do I try and control my disgust? Do I complain about ingratitude, and point this out to the sick and their families? And yet only one person cured of leprosy thanked Christ!

16. How do I approach concerns about the life of the unborn? Do I know the exact position of the Church, and do I act in accordance with it, and offer instructions, advice and support to women, in the light of it? Do I have the courage of my convictions to refuse to help in lethal procedures? Do I back down in this respect, fearing for my job and position? Do I make fun of large families? In the case of a threat to the life of the unborn child, have I done everything in my power mindful of the law and prevailing local rulings, to protect and support the unborn child and the welfare of the mother.

17. Do I embrace with special care unmarried mothers, attempting to rekindle their suppressed or misplaced maternal love and assure them proper support and living conditions?

18. Do I foster contempt for "social outcasts", such as alcoholics, young offenders, prostitutes? Do I dismiss them saying, "It's not worth bothering about them?"

Part V

1. What is my relationship with my colleagues: doctors, nurses, allied health professionals and other people in the team in which I work?

2. If I work in an atmosphere of intrigue, envy, laziness, gossip, irresponsibility, and corruption — do I succumb, or on the contrary — do I try to clean it up? Do I exacerbate heated disputes or just the opposite — do I try and mitigate them and create harmony? Do I easily take offense, becoming irritable, petty; and am I unforgiving of slights?

3. Do I realize that as a Catholic my duty is to evangelize, above all by example? On the other hand do I flaunt my zeal and devotion?

4. Maybe among my colleagues are decent people who are however non-religious, while other so-called practicing colleagues are less concerned about the sick and are less conscientious? Am I therefore led astray with temptations against the value of professing my faith?

5. Am I afraid to expose my superiors and colleagues where there is a need to oppose something which interferes with the good of the patient? Do I cowardly hide the mistakes of others, and tolerate evil? Do I tolerate someone else's dishonesty through a mistaken belief in collegiality?

6. Do I maintain the dignity of my profession in regard to doctors? Do I try and encourage patients to respect medical authority?

7. Do I willingly stand-in for my colleagues when necessary, without mentioning favors; have I visited sick colleagues, and shown them compassion for their misfortune? Am I trustworthy and mindful of other people's time? Do they wait for me in vain?

8. What is my attitude towards novice colleagues who are just beginners? Do I dampen their enthusiasm or lower the standard of work? Do I help them, sharing with them my experiences; am I understanding of their needs? What is my attitude towards nurses and personnel with lower qualifications than me? Do I show them disrespect, discouraging them from their assigned work, forgetting that all work is equally important, because it all serves the sick? Do I care about my colleagues' continuing education?

9. What is my attitude towards the non-professional staff? Am I sufficiently demanding but at the same time polite and kind; am I a good role model for them by my conscientiousness and diligence?

10. If I am in a responsible position — do I set a good example by working with the sick, when time permits me? Am I quite demanding, or am I too lax, worried about my popularity? Have I given up trying to raise the professional and moral standards of nurses? Do I shut myself in my office not wanting to know or think about what's going on — in which case why am I there? Do I care enough about the welfare of my staff?

Transcript of talk delivered by Bl. Hanna Chrzanowska
14 February 1973, *in Warsaw, to The Bishops Committee on Pastoral Care*

Lay Apostolate and Care of the Sick

I represent parish care of the sick that is, Parish Nursing, which is part of the ministry of the Archdiocese of Kraków for the sick, infirm and disabled.

What I have to say — I will say in the name of Parish Nurses, both lay and religious, based on our nearly 16 year experience. The underlying philosophy of our work from its very inception had a religious character; that is, to help those who are suffering to carry their Cross, and through them to help Christ. It cannot be otherwise, because after all, our work came into being as work of the Church. From the very beginning we tried to seek inspiration for our work from the pages of the Gospels, where there are so many examples of Christ's relationship with those who are suffering... Overcoming a lot of difficulties we managed to set up our work in most of the Kraków parishes and in a large number of towns in the diocese. The statistics that have been recently completed covering the span of time till the end of 1971, show that we have looked after 2,625 patients. This may seem to be a rather small number, but this statistic includes also those patients who have been nursed from the very beginning. At that time there were only several patients not the six hundred which we have now. We have not prepared the statistics for the year 1972 yet, as this work is arduous and time-consuming, since we prepare the statistics exactly and honestly, yet in the hierarchy of our many tasks, this is not considered that important.

We work according to the Statutes of Parish Nursing, and I will briefly present here the rules of this regulation, since we closely follow them in our work.

1. A parish nurse is a parish employee, hired and paid for by the parish-priest. Payment is for professional work and the fulfilment of her duties, which demand full time employment, and this differentiates her from other parish workers, although like them, she is a full member of the parish team. However the payment does not negate the charity aspect her of work, nor does it diminishes this aspect of her work. The parish nurse acts on behalf of the parish-priest, taking care of all the chronically ill and old people. She works with such patients as those with rheumatism, paralysis, patients suffering from cancer, indeed anyone who it can be said to have been touched by the hand of Christ. In other words, all the sick who need nursing care.

2. Parish nursing is not only nursing care of the poor. It is not the material status of a patient but a true necessity of nursing care that is the criterion for accepting patients. Neither is it our task to care for specifically lonely people or those who feel lonely. Patients can have a family, even be living together with relatives, but they are working outside of the home, or are also infirm themselves, or they may simply have no idea how to go about nursing a relative. Parish nurses do not work in eight hour shifts, nor do they take on night duties - they spend with their patients as much time as is necessary with each patient. That is why each of the nurses can work with an average of six patients a day, however the overall number can be much larger, as not all the patients require daily nursing visits but only systematic nursing. The sick are nursed regardless of their political or religious views and in spite of the state of the patient's environment. The parish nurses are either qualified professional nurses, or people especially prepared for the work, on three-month courses which are organised every year by The Council for Women Religious of the Diocese of Kraków. Thanks to that our parish nurses not only know how to nurse, but can also assess the social context of the patient, which helps them to decide whether, and to what extent a given patient should be nursed. Generally, nursing sisters work as our parish nurses and through this apostolate some religious congregations manage to fulfil their apostolic mission. I must add, that co-operation between lay nurses and nursing sisters (whose number is much larger), is very good, one could say almost perfect. There is also the issue that the sisters' habit increases her authority in

the eyes of the sick. The sisters' habit invokes confidence, and the sick are convinced, that the nursing care which the sisters extend over them is really reliable. Of course, there is also the potential danger of institutionalisation, as we do not want wish parish nurses to be the only group who nurse the sick. On the contrary, we try to create and focus around ourselves various lay organisations who are fulfilling extremely valuable apostolates.

3. We also try to organise neighbourly help. It sometimes happens that somebody will telephone me with a complaint that neighbours are taking care of someone who is ill. They ask me, "Why doesn't a parish nurse go in there - and I answer, why shouldn't a neighbour go in there if he is willing and able to do so... It is not our intention to detract from the normal expression of neighbourly love either among family members or among neighbours. We all know, that in Poland the process of secularisation is becoming wider and wider and the State Health Service is no exception here. Even if there are believers among its staff, people who are true Catholics, they can only make a difference in their immediate surrounding, without any possibilities of effecting much wider change.

The Health Service itself, although theoretically very noble, has no means of putting into practice its noble ideals. If only the state Health Service provided the chronically ill with adequate nursing care in their own homes. Unfortunately, this is only a dream. The Red Cross auxiliary nurses do visit the sick in their homes, as well as social workers, but in fact the so called trained public health nurses have so many other assignments that the proper nursing care of patients in their homes gets lost somewhere in all their activities. I do not disregard the efforts of the State, but in this situation it can be clearly seen how the words of psalm are fulfilled: "If the Lord will not build a house, useless are the builder's efforts." The reason is that all those people trained how to care for the chronically ill and /or old people on Red Cross nursing courses and are not given any spiritual foundations, but only well-developed professional knowledge. I must add, based on our experiences from Kraków, that parish nursing outstrips any of the work done by the Red Cross home units, and that the number of patients requiring our help does not get any smaller. It must also be added that the Red Cross auxiliary nurses only take care of the sick for specified period of time and not like us till the very end of a patient's life. So what to do with the chronically ill house - bound patient? Such an attitude is sadly characteristic of purely secular activities. On the other hand we nurse some patients over many years. There are many who have been nursed by us for a year or even three or five years and we have other patients whom we have nursed for over ten years.

4. It is self-evident, that nursing an ill person on behalf of the Church cannot be restricted to purely physical nursing activities; it has to also have some apostolic character. From the very beginning we have attempted to follow the words of Pope Pius XII from his Encyclical about The Mystical Body of Christ -"Priesthood among those who are sick lies not only in the hands of anointed priests, but among all those, who perform acts of charity towards the sick." Issues associated with this form of apostolate have also been discussed in the Council documents (which have been so clearly presented to us by our chaplain). We try to deliver our nursing care of the sick at the highest possible (professional) level, but simultaneously we are developing our work in this other [spiritual] direction. In truth it is impossible to speak about two directions, as there is only one direction, because a person is one psychosomatic unite. After all, we have a very strong confirmation of this in the Gospel: "A glass of water given in the name of Christ..." words full of love. "Give her something to eat". The treatment of infirm bodies and through that the healing of ill souls, these are truly gospel activities, which deepen our understanding about the psychosomatic unity of man.

5. We did not dare to predict the full extent of the consequences of our work, even in the area that is after all the essence of our lay apostolate among the sick, in spite of the fact that it came into being from a religious motivation. That is, the conversion of non-believers and the deepening of faith of believers and attempting to bring about the situation when, a person in the course of their illness is ready to say "Yes" to God. The work we do, the kind of services we deliver, is an apostolate of action, not words, and this helps in preparing the way [for conversion]. How can a suffering man comprehend the depth of Christianity, or even an aspect of Christianity, when he is unwell and

neglected, and cannot see any effort being made to bring him physical relief? After all we deal with people who are chronically ill, who often suffer terribly.

We can often prevent that suffering just by good nursing care and sometimes even manage to partially restore their independence. Such interventions are extremely difficult in most typical household conditions. They require a lot of experience and inventiveness. It should be added that parish nurses often work in really terrible conditions even in the apparently comfortable apartment mansions in the centre of the city. I must mention here, that most priests even those working among the sick on behalf of the parish are not aware of these conditions. This is nothing strange, since great cleaning starts as soon as it is heard that a priest is about to visit the household (and it should be like that, in order to show respect towards the priest and Him in whose name he comes). I remember the time when I had the honour of accompanying the Cardinal (Karol Wojtyła) as he was visiting the sick and I wanted to show him some of the terrible living conditions of our patients. And what did we find? Everything was covered with sheets of white paper! He simply saw nothing, and one could not even start to imagine what was going on there. Well, it sometimes happens like that.

6. It should be remembered, that the suffering of a chronically ill person is independent of his material status, or his standard of living. Meanwhile spiritual needs remain the same, and neglect in this sphere is sometimes greater among rich people or those from the so-called intelligentsia, than among simple folk. In order to realistically ground the apostolate among the chronically sick, it would be useful to describe for you here the psyche of these people. But generalisations usually create the danger of pigeonholing, which in turn makes it difficult to perceive each patient as a separate individual. However there are some common features, which can be pointed out. I want to discuss them briefly for you basing my observations on my own experiences, as they are very closely connected with our apostolate. I will not deal here with the problems of psycho - pathology neither the care of psychiatric patients nor with the problem of old people with psychiatric disturbances, as these constitute a completely different problem. I want to speak about the average chronically ill patient.

7. The presence of chronic disease causes the patient to concentrate on them self. Patients are forced by their illness and pain, which is greater or smaller, less or more immobilising to become isolated from the external world, alone in their flat, spending all their time surrounded by the same people, which is often a very narrow group of people. The sick in effect become increasingly isolated. Such a situation is the reason for their growing egocentrism, which we perceive as a natural phenomenon, and nothing surprising. It is almost inevitable that the "ego" of a chronically sick person is more dominant than in any of us. Chronically ill patients are totally dependent on the efforts of people that surround them. Often they cannot properly estimate the strength and endurance of people who are helping them. They keep increasing their demands. They stop understanding other people and that is often the cause of much conflict, in which by no means, one can say that the patient is always right, not at all. Every person desires freedom and also a sick person looks for freedom. And that is the reason for their constant fight with their infirm bodies and that fight brings with it the feeling of rebellion. They are obsessed with the feeling of uselessness. It is also a great worry for those, for whom their illness allows them only to help a little around the house; this is even the case among those who can earn some money working at home.

I would like to mention here that work offered to our patients by different co-operatives completely does not take into account the psychological aspect of labour and sometimes the work is extremely tiring because of its monotony, not to speak of how badly it is paid. All the sick - young and old - have a sense of their human dignity and this should be respected. Especially young disabled people want to be treated normally. For them their physical anomaly is their norm. They are sometimes intellectually very active, and full of interest in life. Under an apparent apathy, life in them often simply vibrates. They cannot stand experiencing so-called pity, staring at them, and asking them questions. Older patients do not want to be treated as children -" sinking into a second childhood" - this is not an appropriate expression, to tell the truth, it refers only to aspects of their physical care, which these people need, but not to their individuality. Indeed they bring with themselves the burden of their whole life. Most chronically ill patients have excellent powers of observation and they are often very critical not only of their families and associates, but of parish workers, priests included.

8. I have only briefly touched on the problem of the sick person's psyche, referring only to those areas which should be familiar to a parish nurse and every parish worker; and generally to every person, who has any contact with the sick. In delivering nursing care, it is necessary to take into consideration the psyche of the chronically ill patient, as one cannot limit oneself to what is universally called, charity regarding the soul and body. In our case we care for the infirm body and through this nursing intervention create the possibility for a close relationship between the patient and God. It is necessary to offer the sick person everything that he or she may need for healthy living. To widen their horizons by delivering to them entertainment, such as good literature, and this does not necessarily mean spiritual reading, [!] to assure them of companionship from outside of their everyday circle, e.g. from among other parish workers, youth and even children. And what about summer holidays, day-trips for our patients, etc. What blessed relaxation! Or an organised retreat which besides the important religious aspect also offers the patient rest and the companionship of other [new] people - such actions give really huge beneficial results. It is wrong to see in a patient only a suffering individual, and not a normal person harbouring their own dreams and desires. However, going back to the nature of our lay apostolate, as that is the main topic of my exposé, we must add here, that we who nurse the sick are in the best of positions due to the very nature of our work – this systematic service to the infirm – to clear the way to their souls.

9. Once we nursed an old gentleman, a philosophising mathematician, who was often visited by priests, but who did not want to receive the sacraments. Yet we still nursed him. After some time he himself said that looking on our work, he could see that the philosophy of Kant was different from the philosophy of the Gospel. Finally, acquiescing to the request of a young nursing sister, who was looking after him, he converted and received the sacraments. There was another patient, in his sixties, introduced to us by a friend of his, not so much to be nursed as to be converted. As it later transpired the gentleman had never

received any sacraments in his life. Well, maybe in his childhood. He was a very intelligent and good man. The need for nursing was great and urgent in his case – a serious neurological disease. His legs were covered in wounds, which quickly healed when they were regularly washed. He found out about our retreats, which take place every year and which are organised by the priests in the Retreat House of Fathers of The Divine Saviour, (Salvatorians) in Trzebinia. He decided to go there, and we cosseted him in the same way as the others, in accordance with the medieval dictum, *Our Masters - the Sick*. He listened to the talks, and took part in all the services. It was very rewarding for us, that he was present with us, but his friend was disappointed, because our gentleman still did not decide to receive the sacraments. However, he had made the first steps. Meanwhile, he was constantly being visited, constantly, I cannot stress this strongly enough, by the retreat master who had made friends with him. As the life of the old gentleman was not threatened, the priest did not hurry, and did not persuade him into doing anything. He simply waited till the desire of this man would awaken. And we were still nursing him… After several months our patient declared that "he wanted to receive the sacraments." I will never forget the expression on his face as he waited for confession and the first Holy Communion in his adult life. He received it during a Mass, celebrated in his own home.

We could multiply such examples endlessly. And the common factor in these acts of conversion is the prayer of the parish nurse. One of our sisters prayed all night and implored the mercy of conversion for a very reluctant woman just a day before her death. A fundamental problem in our apostolate is the nature and mystery of suffering. This is very huge problem and it gets more and more difficult, especially with the spread of materialistic consumption in our society. In such an atmosphere, the spirit of sacrifice is undervalued, or even rendered completely incomprehensible. So it is not easy for a contemporary person to understand the purpose of suffering, which is synonymous with sacrifice and renunciation. At the same time I met several people from among parish workers, strong believers and full of goodwill, who have made some basic mistakes. A suffering person cannot be told," You should be glad that you are suffering, Jesus loves you and that is why you suffer". Perhaps, this is the truth, but it cannot reach these people;

quite the opposite it may create a barrier in their relationship with God. Such statements may be understandable to some people, but they cannot be used as a ready-made formula with everyone. Among our patients there is a certain woman in her forties, incurably ill from her childhood. She has a lot of time and intellectual capabilities to think over the problem of suffering. Based on her observations and on our own experience we can assure you, that in most cases the answer to the question "Why me? ", or "What is this for?", is best answered simply, by 'this is God's mystery, in the same way as God's mystery is the Suffering of Christ'.

10. I have noticed, that even a rebellious patient, awaiting discussion on this subject, someone who is full of internal turmoil, yet faced with such a response ceases to discuss, calms down, and becomes more trustful. And this is the foundation upon which other truths will grow, the full truth, the one which will bring liberation to the sick. And the ill need liberation so desperately. They cannot escape the enslavement of their bodies, but they can drop, or at least relax their spiritual fetters. And we in this manner can clear the way for the priest. And we (in Parish Nursing)should all be aware, that we clear the way for the priest.

11. An issue of great importance is the prayer of the sick, which besides its own value can bring them relief in their feeling of uselessness, once they understand the redeeming power of prayer. And here too we should be extremely careful in our apostolate. We mustn't force our favourite forms of prayer on our patients. There was a situation when a parish worker forced a seriously ill woman to recite the whole rosary. As a result of this the ill woman did not want to have anything to do with anybody from the parish.

I will never forget a personal experience which 1 had when I was working in a hospital and I overheard a conversation between two patients. One of them said to the other "I am no longer able to even say the 'Our Father', I am not able to even say a 'Hail Mary', I only say 'My God' and I think, that the Lord understands such abbreviations." I will never forget that. We all know that the aim of our lay apostolate among the sick is to help them to convert and to deepen their faith. But we, whether secular nurses or religious sisters, should be very careful concerning '*the deepening of faith,*' so as not to act like "predacious wolves, or false prophets."

First of all we must be humble. We are not in a position to understand completely the nature of suffering, to feel the pain caused by long immobilisation; we do not know what really happens in the soul of an ill person. We mustn't lord over them, we must only serve. Otherwise we would not be following the example of Christ. We cannot go to our patients with the conviction that we will raise them to some spiritual heights. Whose? Ours? God help us! Don't delude yourselves, that we will inevitably deepen their faith. Very often the situation is quite the opposite, it is they who deepen our faith and enrich us. It is precisely those silent and meek patients, who manage to keep to themselves their 'holiest of holy spaces in their innermost soul." Like the young girl suffering from cancer, dying fully conscious, offering her life for morally lost youth. The young boy completely immobilised by rheumatism, who radiates an inner life, without saying a word; or another young boy with muscular dystrophy, who read once in a periodical that people were sending parcels to the missions, but he did not have any money to send, so he asked us to let them know, that he will be praying for [the work of] the missions. When compared with such people, we are useless servants in accordance with the words of St. Luke.

12. We very often meet with a lot of difficulties surrounding the sacrament of Extreme Unction [Sacrament of the Sick and the Last Rites]. Much time will need to elapse before people will forget about superstitions connected with this sacrament and before the priest will not be seen as a herald of death. The proper way in which the sacrament of Extreme Unction should be perceived, as it was presented to us during the Council, will not become popular for a long time to come. I must add, that during our retreats one of our priests offers this sacrament to every person, who asks for it. And this is the best way of teaching people, of increasing their knowledge about this sacrament. Everybody participates in this pious act — the old and the young — in public in the presence of everyone gathered in the chapel. On the subject of Holy Sacraments, it is necessary to stress the fact, that when an ill person is preparing to be admitted to hospital they should try and

receive the sacraments at home… We all know what the situation in hospitals is like. Therefore it is one of our greatest duties to ensure for the patients the possibility of receiving the sacraments [in the privacy of their homes].

13. We are dealing here with the problem of death. According to our statistics, there have been 1110 patient deaths. These figures are not terrifying, on the contrary, it is a great honour for us, that thanks to the care of parish workers we could help such a large number of people in their pilgrimage to Our Father's house. The eschatological dimension of our work can be fully appreciated in these figures. It is not just the lack of this eschatological appreciation among the faithful that makes for the proper attitude to approaching death so difficult for the sick and their families. The fact that we ourselves, at least as long as we are healthy, are not afraid of death that is quite another matter. However, it does not mean, that we do not acknowledge the fact of the fear of death existing among our patients. Such fears exist and are quite natural. The fact that most patients hold on so desperately to the thin thread of life is on one hand proof of their having been brought-up without adequate understanding of death, but on the other hand it demonstrates how precious the gift of life is to everyone. How strongly old people fight for their life - the question: "Am I dying?" is quite frequent. And such questions should be answered individually. Not everyone is given the gift and rare mercy of facing death eye to eye with defiance: Such as the "ars *moriendi*" (trans.: the gift of dying), which was given to the late Teresa Strzembosz. At times like that we can only behave with tact and respect.

14. It is one thing to proffer trivial consolation and something quite different to answer carefully and gently so as not to cause shock. Hypocrites' "*primum non nocere*" (trans: Above all do no harm) has here one of its best applications. It seems advisable to follow the advice of a priest who works closely with us: do not attempt to console, but simply answer: "that nobody knows who is to die first – neither you nor me." We will all die one day, and I would add from myself here, fortunately. Of course everything depends on the patient's personality. And yet, in spite of our deep faith concerning the presence of everlasting happiness in Our Lord's house, we still treat the family of someone who has

just lost someone with all our compassion. Assurances about prayer and real sincerity only exceptionally can be substituted for religious conversations so soon after the death of someone close. Most importantly, it is necessary to beware of all triviality.

A close acquaintance of mine, who lost her little boy, left the Church after assurances from friends about a little angel in heaven. We must respect human pain. We must respect the 'Mater Dolorosa'. But it must also be said, that if someone dies at home, he is really lucky. We know what death in a hospital looks like – often somewhere behind a screen, without care, or even in a corridor. Even in institutions, where nursing sisters' work – a long drawn-out agony in a shared room provokes aggression among other patients. General insensibility to the suffering of others and the general lack of sensibility to somebody's death is quite common. We must avoid useless talking while someone is dying. I witnessed once a situation, where a patient was still breathing, and people were already looking over her desk for money. Our role is great here. We must teach people how to pray at the bedside of the dying and of course, we ourselves must pray, though naturally not necessarily on our knees, but definitely not neglecting our duties. I do not want to claim, by any means, that apostolic work among the sick – that is – converting and deepening the faith of patients and clearing the way for the priest, can be done only by the parish nurses, and not by any other parish worker.

Everything that I have said applies anyone who has any contact with the sick, although I fully realise that our task is made easier. After all, there are a large number of people in the parishes, who do not need our nursing care, because they have it guaranteed by somebody else, but still even these parishioners should have some contact with their parish through parish workers. However, even among those people who are nursed by us, visits from outside of the nursing staff are very desirable, especially visits from parish helpers, but always working in agreement with the parish nurse. We can observe among many of our patients, even those considering themselves to be religious, a kind of religious illiteracy. There are many homes without a copy of the Bible. People need to be prepared to celebrate the Holy Mass at home. After all, these are people, who did not receive any instructions concerning post-conciliar teachings about lay participation in the Mass. Yet these are activities for which a parish nurse has usually very little time. However, any person undertaking this kind of work should act with great gentleness and integrity. We must also always be prepared, that the patient may be operating on a much higher spiritual level than ourselves. And what about a nursing sister? She should closely cooperate in her apostolic work with the parish priest. I say sincerely that "she should", because this co-operation is not always possible. It is often limited to asking the priest to come to visit the sick, or to fix a date for giving out Holy Communion, or arranging a date to celebrate Mass ; that is, to the most basic matters.

15. We rejoice very much, that we can be the link between the ill person and the priest where the problem of holy sacraments is concerned, as they are the only true way to Our Lord. On the other hand, the words of Father Wiesen, a Camillian priest, whom I read not long ago, *"We must not forget that there is still a very long way to go from receiving the sacraments to a truly Christian acquiescence to disease and infirmity,"* are really very true. Often priests limit their visits to the sick to distributing the sacraments and religious matters. It happened not so long ago that one of our parish nurses asked a priest to visit one of her patients, who was having spiritual problems. The priest thought that he should go with the Holy Sacraments and was very displeased, when the patient refused to receive the Sacraments.

Similar situations take place, at least according to our reports, in other large urban parishes. There is quite a different situation in small parishes, where the parish-priest and his assistants know their flock. I understand perfectly well, the problems of pastoral work in large parishes, but if a parish nurse asks for help with a difficult case, her request should not go unheeded. The situation is similar when the priest's presence is asked for in other non-urgent cases, and where it ought to be part of the priest's regular visits to the homes of parishioners, in order to support them. In some large parishes there is a special priest, whose task it is to serve the sick and infirm. It is no business of mine to judge whether such specialisation is good in every case. I dare only to ask, whether depriving other priests of the opportunity to visit the sick does not detract something from their pastoral duties? Each specialisation has its strong and weak points.

16. Co-operation of parish nurses with parish priests should be char-acterised by great mutual openness. The parish nurse should consult with the priest about ways of dealing with her patients, and present the patient's problems to him for discussion. For his part the priest should help by pointing out to the parish nurse how she can solve the problem. As I have already mentioned, sick people especially young ones and so called intellectuals can be very critical.

It often happens that such a person, having every day contact with his or her parish nurse and trusting her, informs her about his/her impressions and feelings. Ill people hate clichés of any kind. They want to see the priest as their friend, someone with whom they can share their sorrows and problems and simultaneously they want to be treated normally, in the same way as healthy people. I remember one young boy with rheumatoid arthritis, who was at the threshold of conversion, who upon being taken to church for a regular public Mass, said: "At last I did not have to listen to a sermon about disease and suffering, but an ordinary sermon about God." Some patients do not want to listen to what they call "preaching," that is, a priest's mono-logue. And they do not want to listen about suffering because they are not always ready to accept its deepest sense.

17. The Holy Mass at home, this really wonderful celebration, can sometimes become a torment for the sick person, if it lengthens too much as a result of a long homily, or protracted recitation of commu-nal bidding prayers and thanksgiving. After the Mass some patients wish to stay silent and say their own prayers in concentration. Others, although very religious, refuse to take part in the Mass, because this excites them too much nervously.

Religious slides do not always deepen spirituality, because such shows may make the patient nervous, especially when they take place in the evenings; they can cause insomnia for some patients. We often come across spiritual problems among people from the patients' imme-diate surroundings. Partly because we go to families with very different social backgrounds, and sometimes even to those who do not want to hear about a priest's visit to their home. We often meet Catholic patients who do not want to express their faith as they are afraid of negative reactions from people in their communities. We also go and nurse in crime-infested environments. We cannot refuse anyone. In such situations we must try to be maximally tactful, and we should be cunning in the way that it is described in the Gospel.

Unfortunately, there are more and more of such situations at this time of de-Christianisation in our society. Poor lost people. We can only fulfil our apostolic task witnessing with our actions, without many words. And here again we can observe the influence of our work on the environment of our patients. We know about cases, where thanks to persistent, systematic nursing, not only the hearts of the sick soften, but also of those people in their immediate surrounding. And even if their hearts do not soften can we complain? Surely not! We are simply witnesses of Christ. And that's enough.

You may ask about the benefits that our work brings to the parish; here they are:

- Realisation of one of the parish's main duties - i.e. actively demonstrating love towards the sick and infirm.

- Penetration into many different social environments, which without parish nursing input would remain unknown to the parish; in some cases environments negatively positioned toward Christ and the Church.

- Concentrating together people of goodwill, for example various groups of parish helpers, including young people and children. These groups are extremely valuable [in the promotion of our project], but a description of their work and achievements goes beyond the topic of my already too long speech. And I have already spoken about [the benefits resulting from] mutual relations between priests and parish nurses.

Finally, I beg of you one last thing, may the priests present please not show pity towards us, telling us what a wonderful work we are doing, (what a terribly unsuitable expression that is), by fulfilling the lowest services for the sick and disabled, "since there is nothing pleasant in literally smearing your fingers in ...." We are happy we can serve in this way; and besides can we ever speak about a hierarchy of services when we are helping an unfortunate person? It is so often forgotten, that when Christ gave us His New Commandment he illustrated it with the example of the Good Samaritan. If we follow this precedence, why should we be pitied?

Translated by M. Brykczyńska

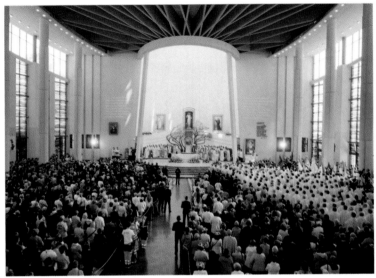

Marie Romagnano

Beatification was attended by hundreds of priests, nurses, other healthcare professionals, laity, dignitaries and the sick.

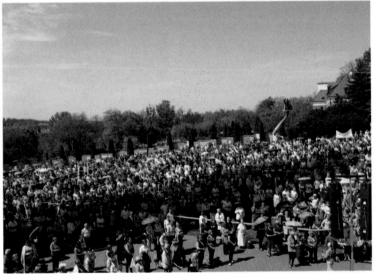

Sisters of Our Lady of Mercy

Crowds outside the Basilica of Divine Mercy in Łagiewniki during the beatification April 28, 2018

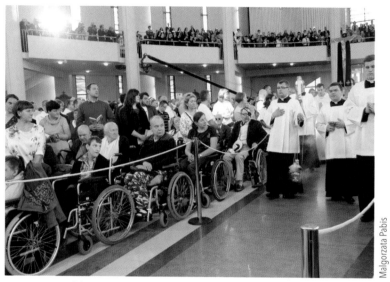

The wheelchair patients are the true VIPs at the
Beatification Ceremony.

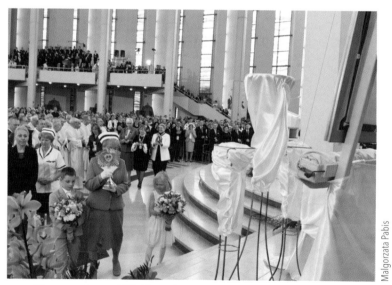

Vice-postulator of Bl. Hanna's canonization cause with a specially
commissioned reliquary by Polish nurses.

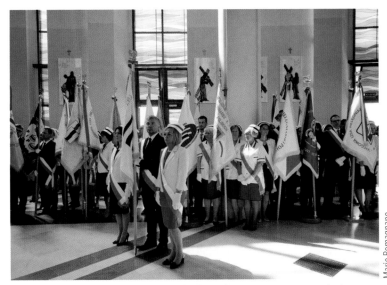

Nurses from around Poland at the Beatification ceremony with their school/university banners.

Marie Romagnano

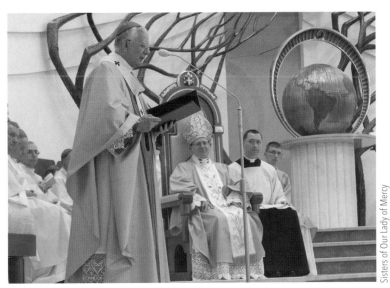

Marek Jędraszewski, Archbishop of Kraków, petitioning Angelo Cardinal Amato S.D.B., Prefect of the Congregation for the Causes of Saints, to beatify Hanna Chrzanowska.

Sisters of Our Lady of Mercy

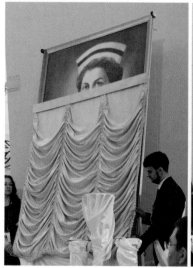
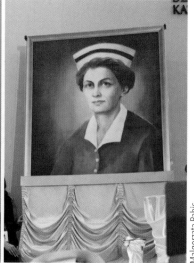

Unveiling the Beatification portrait of Blessed Hanna

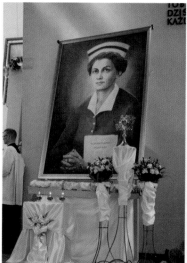
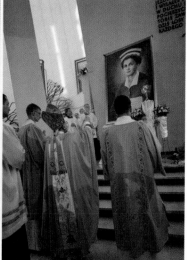

Left: Beatification picture and reliquary and three lit lamps placed
there by nurses representing the worldwide nursing community.
Right: Cardinal Amato incensing image of Blessed Hanna.

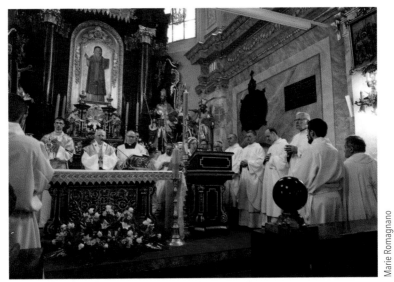

Marie Romagnano

Krystyna Pęchalska of the Association of Catholic Nurses in Kraków reading during the Thanksgiving Mass in St Nicholas' Church for the beatification of Bl. Hanna.

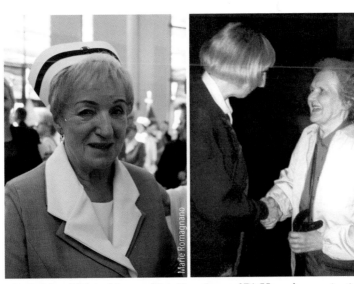

Marie Romagnano

Collection of the author

Left: Mme Helena Matoga, Vice-Postulator of Bl. Hanna's canonization cause, after the beatification ceremony. Bl. Hanna had been her nurse tutor. Right: Author with Alina Rumun, RN who worked the closest with Bl. Hanna on the Parish Nursing project.

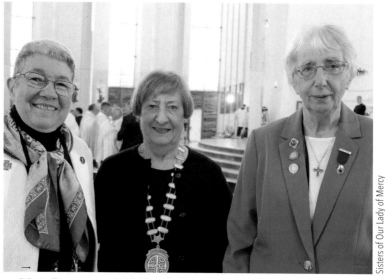

Marie Romagnano, RN, Founder Healthcare Professionals for Divine Mercy, USA; Geraldine McSweeney, RN, President of CICIAMS, Ireland and Dr Gosia Brykczyńska, RN from United Kingdom.

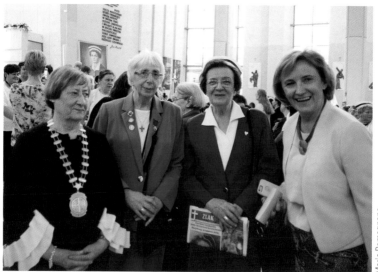

First from Left - Geraldine McSweeney, President of CICIAMS; Dr Gosia Brykczyńska, author; Mme Krystyna Wolska-Lipiec, Chair of the History of Nursing Society of the Polish Nursing Association (PTP); Dr Grażyna Wójcik, President of the Polish Nurses Association (PTP)

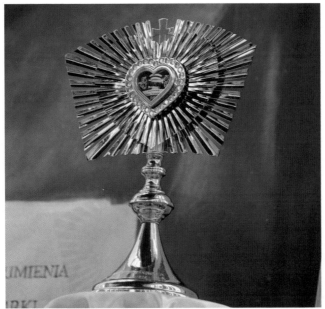

Specially commissioned reliquary in the shape of a heart, by the Polish nurses, containing relics of Bl. Hanna. Note the miniature nurses cap…

Marie Romagnano

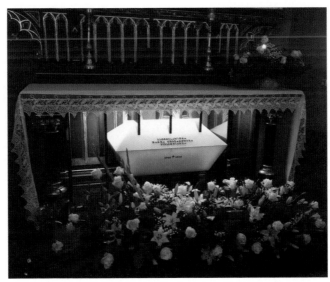

Alabaster sarcophagus with the mortal remains of Bl Hanna in St Nicholas' Church.

Marie Romagnano

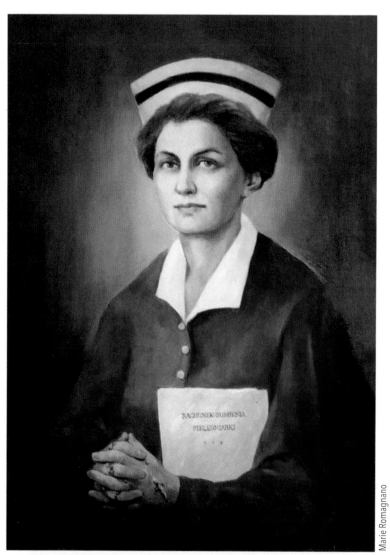

Beatification portrait of Bl. Hanna Chrzanowska holding the
Nurses Examination of Conscience.